migraine *expressions*

A Creative Journey through Life with Migraine

Compiled and Edited by Betsy Baxter Blondin

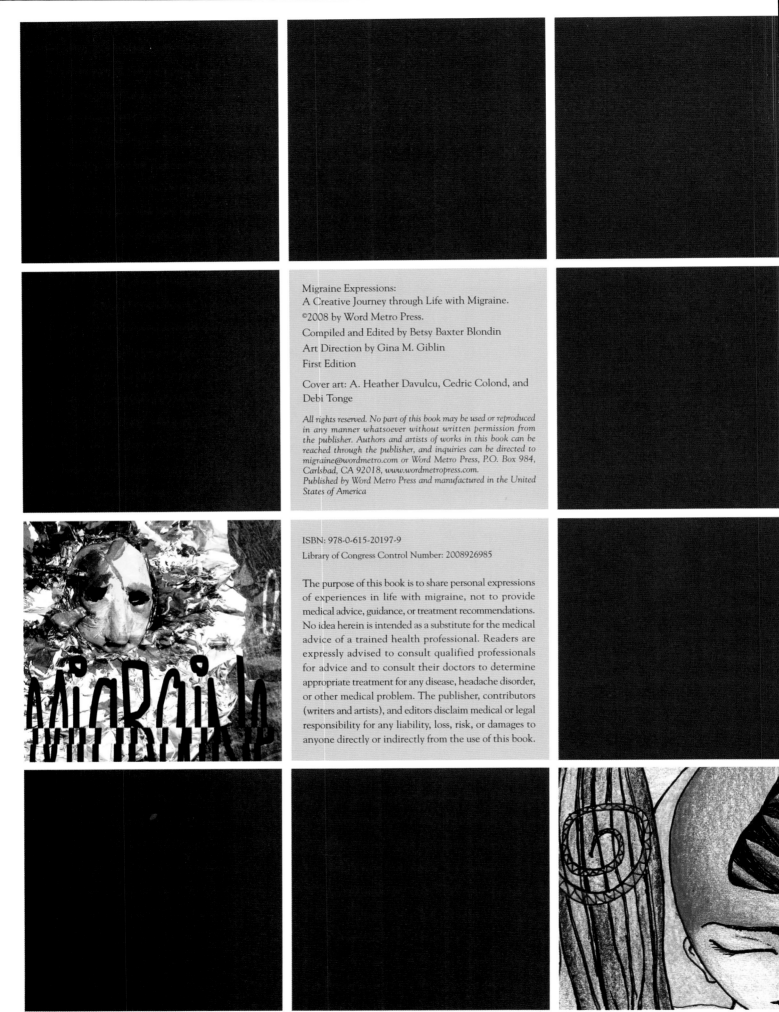

Migraine Expressions:
A Creative Journey through Life with Migraine.
©2008 by Word Metro Press.
Compiled and Edited by Betsy Baxter Blondin
Art Direction by Gina M. Giblin
First Edition

Cover art: A. Heather Davulcu, Cedric Colond, and Debi Tonge

ISBN: 978-0-615-20197-9
Library of Congress Control Number: 2008926985

The purpose of this book is to share personal expressions of experiences in life with migraine, not to provide medical advice, guidance, or treatment recommendations. No idea herein is intended as a substitute for the medical advice of a trained health professional. Readers are expressly advised to consult qualified professionals for advice and to consult their doctors to determine appropriate treatment for any disease, headache disorder, or other medical problem. The publisher, contributors (writers and artists), and editors disclaim medical or legal responsibility for any liability, loss, risk, or damages to anyone directly or indirectly from the use of this book.

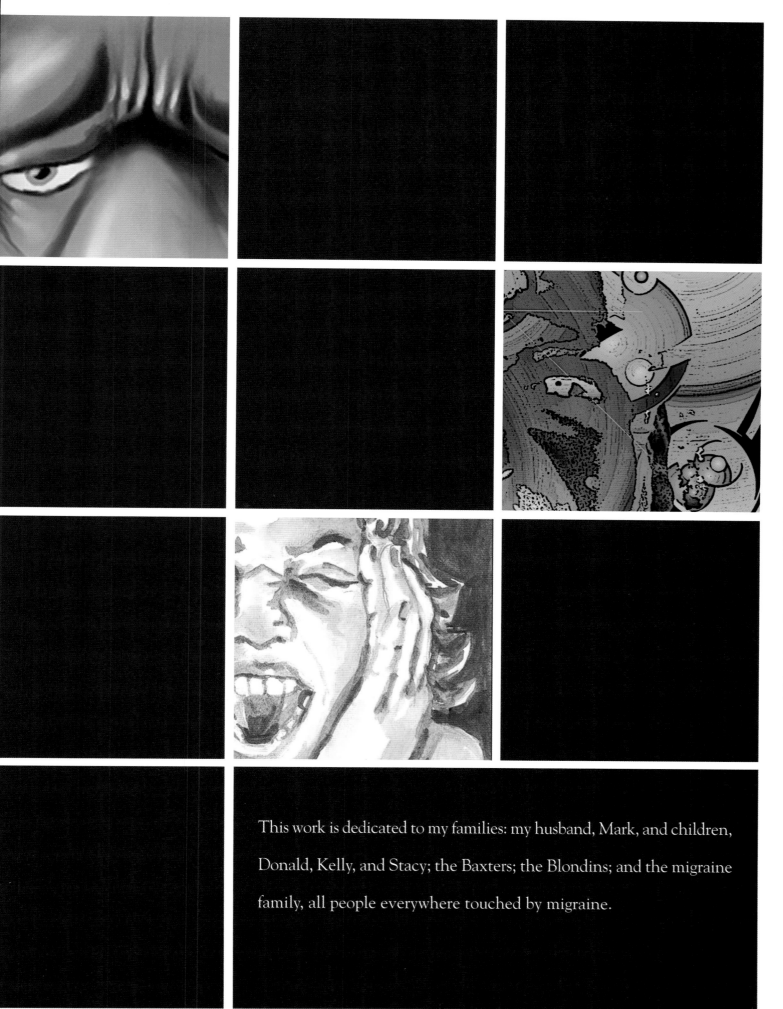

This work is dedicated to my families: my husband, Mark, and children, Donald, Kelly, and Stacy; the Baxters; the Blondins; and the migraine family, all people everywhere touched by migraine.

acknowledgements

My dream for this book became a reality because of the migraine expressions and support I received from so many in the worldwide migraine family; I am deeply grateful for that, and…

…To the hundreds of individuals living with migraine who shared their courageous and insightful work, and just as importantly their offers of help, validating comments, and friendship. With special thanks to Melissa Bartosh for her valuable assistance and enthusiasm.

…To the many migraine professionals and headache organization staff who provided feedback, ideas, and assistance in promoting the project, including Teri Robert, Ph.D., author, educator, and patient advocate, and Andrew M. Blumenfeld, M.D., who both also reviewed content for me; Suzanne Simons, Executive Director of the National Headache Foundation; and Karen Manning of the Migraine Action Association.

…To the bloggers who posted or allowed me to post notices on their sites and or sent creative material for the book, including Teri Robert of My Migraine Connection, Health Central Network, Ronda Solberg of The Migraine Page, Kerrie Smyres of The Daily Headache, Jackie Taylor of Life in the Canadian Desert, and James Cottrill of Relieve Migraine Headache.

…To others who by simply sending encouraging comments inspired me to keep working in spite of my own challenges, including all those who submitted materials, Scott Madden of the Michigan Head-Pain & Neurological Institute, Larry Robbins, M.D., of the Robbins Headache Clinic, Brent Lucas of Help for Headaches, and countless others who know they helped.

…And of course to my family for their help with all aspects of this project, including their creative contributions – but most of all for their love and faith in me.

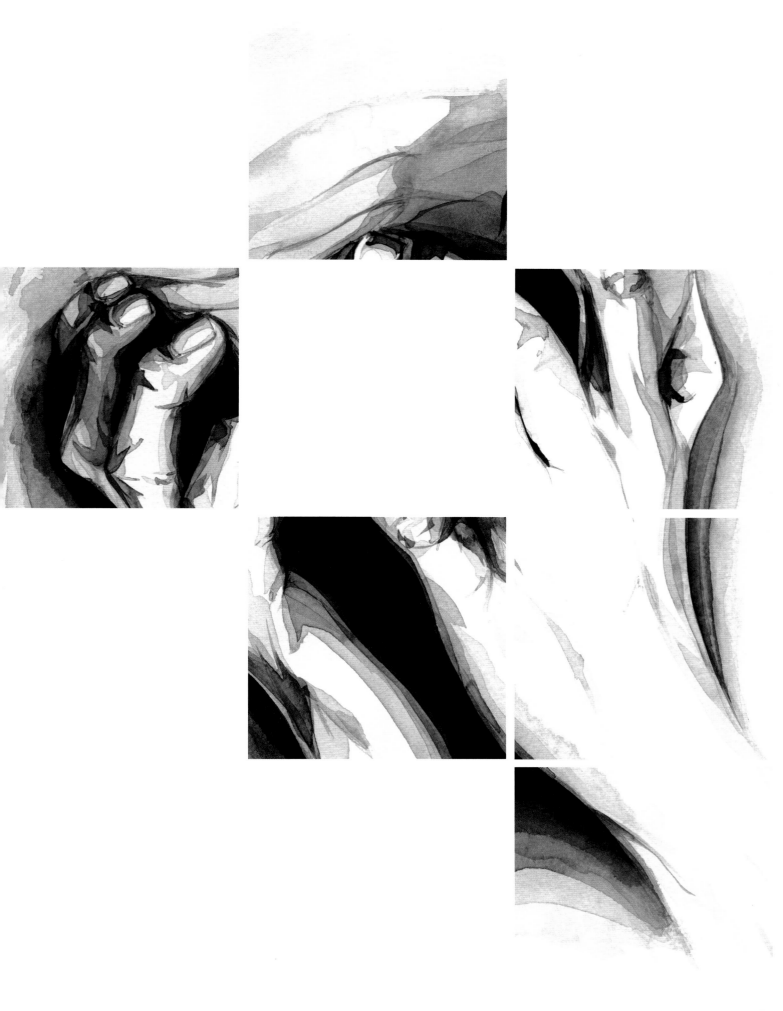

mi·graine

Pronunciation: mI-grAn, Brit often mE-grAn
Function: noun

◆genetic, neurological disease, sometimes referred to as a neurobiological disorder: symptoms include recurring episodes or attacks of throbbing head pain, usually severe, typically but not always on one side and aggravated by physical activity; nausea; vomiting; abdominal pain; increased sensitivity to light, sounds and or smells; and possibly diarrhea, dizziness, fatigue, blurred vision, and scalp pain

◆symptoms and frequency of attacks, which do not always include head pain, vary for each individual; attacks can last from two hours to three days, sometimes longer

◆caused by neurological (physical), not psychological, factors

◆one of the primary headache disorders; others are tension and cluster headache

◆several types of migraine exist, without aura and with aura (visual disturbances) being the most common

IMPORTANT: *Seek medical help if you have a combination of these or similar symptoms.*

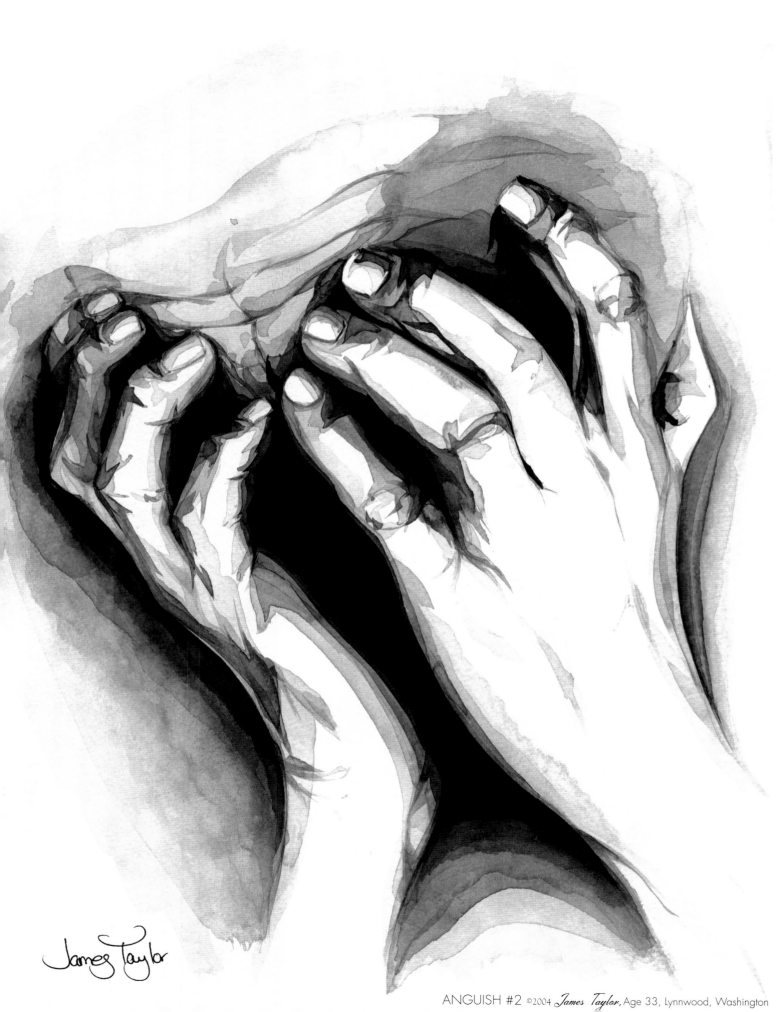

James Taylor

ANGUISH #2 ©2004 *James Taylor*, Age 33, Lynnwood, Washington

contents

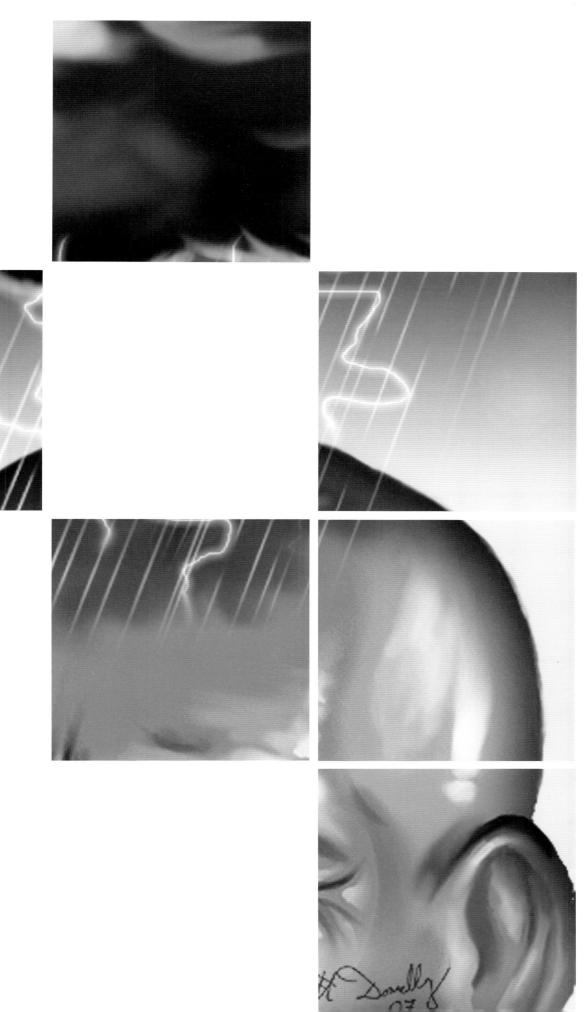

introduction

Betsy Baxter Blondin
May 2008

migraine. It is a world of its own in the universe of primary headache disorders, a neurological disease that debilitates and limits millions of people of all countries, ages, and walks of life. If you think *headache* when you hear the word *migraine*, think again. The following migraine expressions will enlighten you if you're not among the millions who recognize them as too familiar. While *Migraine Expressions* represents a milestone in my personal migraine journey, I hope this book will be meaningful to you and a place you revisit often to discover new insights, whether you are an immediate member of the migraine family, a relative, visitor, or health care giver.

For many years I have wanted to publish a book that would combine written and visual art, providing a platform for creative expressions of people who live with migraine while intrinsically promoting a better understanding of it. The courage and strength it takes to live with migraine, while managing to enjoy families, maintain friendships, earn academic degrees, have successful careers, and sometimes just to get out of bed in the morning is phenomenal. That strength and courage as well as a wealth of talent are apparent in the expressions of pain, fear, and aloneness, hope, optimism, and accomplishments of this representative group of migraineurs.

My first migraine attack struck savagely at age 16 and for many subsequent years I did not know what I had or that there was help for me. In retrospect, I certainly wish I had been more assertive, but instead I hid or downplayed my suffering. The first doctor with whom I discussed my head pain and accompanying symptoms ignorantly advised me to stroke my chin and relax while warning me that I was likely to have an ulcer to go with my "headache" by age 25. This lack of awareness and a widespread attitude toward women and headaches, typical in those years, led me to hide my affliction even more, delaying any meaningful diagnosis or treatment.

For 15 years, I suffered several migraine episodes each month, struggled through school and work, sometimes spending up to three days in bed alternating between vomiting and sleeping, always with pain. And my experiences, I came to learn, were not nearly as bad as those of others! My epiphany occurred when I happened on an illustrated *Smithsonian* magazine article about migraines. With one glance at the artwork, I not only identified what I had but also realized with extreme relief that I was not alone in my terrible experience. Subsequently, an obstetrician I was seeing formally diagnosed my symptoms as migraine and I started on a long path of further discovery, one on which I continue.

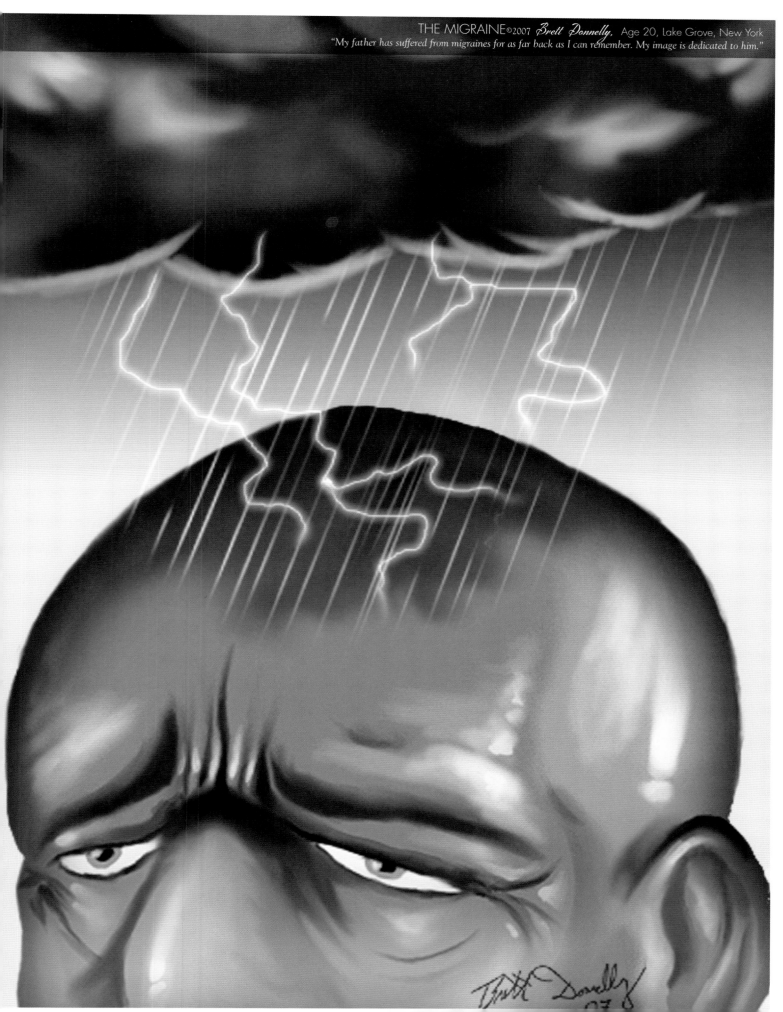

THE MIGRAINE ©2007 *Brett Donnelly*, Age 20, Lake Grove, New York
"My father has suffered from migraines for as far back as I can remember. My image is dedicated to him."

My nearly 40-year trek has led me to the completion of this book, a vantage point from where I can assess my long adventure. I reflect on the last year with pleasure and awe at the stunningly intimate work people from many countries sent, the validating and inspiring insights they shared, and the friends I have found.

While collecting this material, I was astounded, honored, and grateful that so many people impacted by migraine submitted such outstanding visual and written expressions. They confirmed my belief that this book by and from migraineurs will promote understanding among people without migraine and work as a catalyst for advancing awareness, assessment, discussion, research, and development of effective treatments.

At the same time, I was humbled, struck by the extraordinary talent of the people who sent material and by the enormous complexity of migraine and how little I still understood. It quickly became apparent that there are many stages of comprehension; so the book inherently documents the levels of understanding among ourselves, our families, friends, co-workers, and the medical community. Even among experts, knowledge, opinion, and terminology differ, so it is not surprising how challenging it is for migraineurs to grasp the intricacies of migraine and learn how to help ourselves.

Accordingly, I intentionally left intact expressions with which others may not relate or agree. I avoided judging the right or wrong of statements or attempting to edit insights, feelings, and interpretations of individuals' life circumstances. For example, when migraineurs refer to their "migraine headaches," it seems that we can all agree they mean the head pain of a migraine attack, which also includes additional symptoms. Just as migraine research, knowledge, and treatment continue to evolve, each individual's level of migraine knowledge and understanding of their own situation changes. These expressions were created at specific times and exist as snapshots of what migraine feels like and how life can be affected by it.

Likewise, I retained the expressions of frustration with the medical community, the pharmaceutical and insurance industries, and the extreme lack of sufficient research, education, and treatment specifically for migraine. This of course does not mean that helpful, meaningful, and successful medical care does not exist. On the contrary, numerous migraine and headache specialists dedicate their careers to helping people with migraine manage their symptoms and attacks so they can enjoy the best possible quality of life.

You will immediately see and feel what this book *is*, so let me briefly mention what it is not. It is not a medical, informational, or advice book; I am a migraine survivor, patient, and student, not a doctor or migraine expert. The myriad treatments and methods people have employed in their individual efforts to alleviate migraine symptoms, and write about in their work here, are not medical advice. If you have migraine or think you do, or feel you may have a serious headache disorder, I urge you to find an appropriate health care professional, preferably a headache or migraine specialist, be properly diagnosed, educate yourself as much as possible, and exercise patience and diligence in determining how to best manage life with migraine.

The Internet allows us to access current information from migraine organizations, Web sites, blogs, and forums online and benefit from the efforts of committed advocates and health professionals. We can communicate in real time with others who share life with migraine and its challenges. We can compare information about symptoms, medications, alternative treatments, health care professionals, or simply find a sympathetic ear. Included at the end of this book is a list of the helpful migraine organizations, Web sites, and blogs of which I am aware and have often consulted.

Fortunately, tremendous progress has been made toward understanding and treating migraine; no one now needs to suffer in silence as I and many others have. Regrettably, we still have a very long way to go. While this book is intentionally and specifically about life with migraine, more research, education, and awareness are urgently needed for all headache disorders.

Given the magnitude of migraine alone, research is woefully underfunded. One in nine of the world's adults have migraine,[1] and it is among the top 20 causes of healthy life lost to disability.[2] In the United States, the "burden of illness and costs for migraine is greater than that for epilepsy, stroke, Parkinson's disease, multiple sclerosis, and Alzheimer's disease combined!"[3] According to the National Institutes of Health, 21 times more funding is allocated for asthma research than for the study of migraine, even though there are an estimated 36 million people with migraine, 20 million people with asthma, and the annual costs attributable to migraine are 27 times higher than those for asthma. [4] These numbers appear to be comparable per the population in Canada, the UK, and countries of Europe. No one wishes to see research funds decreased for any disease, but rather to see the evident neglect toward migraine research recognized and corrected. While no cure for migraine currently exists, everyone has a real potential for finding effective ways to minimize and control the attacks.

Last year a group of doctors, advocates, and leading headache organizations initiated an effort to convince the U.S. Congress to provide additional funding for research into headache disorders including migraine. This effort culminated in the formation of the Alliance for Headache Disorders Advocacy. See Resources and Advocacy pages for more information on the alliance as well as contact information for the Migraine Research Foundation. If you bought the book you're holding, you have already made a contribution to migraine research advancement efforts via your purchase.

The individuals who sent their work for publication obviously made this book possible. So many people offered so much beautiful and significant material, that it was extremely challenging to select pieces representing various perspectives on aspects of life with migraine. If you submitted writing or art that does not appear in this volume, please know that I remain grateful and honored by your efforts and support; your spirit is indeed part of the book.

While collecting and assembling these works, I was impressed by many things and the following three in particular. First, the gender, ethnicity, age, politics, and professions of contributing individuals were irrelevant because it was only the commonality of migraine among us that mattered. Second, several themes occur in so many creative expressions of

migraine, and I hope you find them as fascinating as I do. And third, no matter how desperate the description, image, symbol, or metaphor in a piece, almost always a tomorrow, a glimpse of hope, or a determination to survive resides there, too.

A few contributors mention the concept of letting go, seeing migraine not as an enemy to battle but as a part of oneself to be accepted and managed; not panicking, acknowledging the pain and releasing negative emotions can make recovery easier. Others speak of a burst of energy or euphoria prior to or at the beginning of a migraine attack, or of trying to comprehend or harness what occurs in the brain during an excruciatingly painful episode. And a majority of us comment on the role that art and writing play in both managing pain and communicating our experience to others when day-to-day conversation fails. After many years of working, writing, and editing for others, between and during migraine episodes, this project has afforded me a year of therapy, a long-awaited and welcomed catharsis. In reflecting on the observation that living with migraine is equivalent to "living loss of life,"[5] I realize that through working on this book with these members of the world's migraine family, I have regained, or at least compensated for, some of my lost life.

There is no comfortable way to make this journey, and many of our expressions are disturbing, tragic, dark, or lonely. That is what living with migraine can be. But there is also humor, light, joy, and hope in these pages — written and visual illustrations of not only our pain but also of our healthy, optimistic, and productive times. These expressions represent everyone around the world touched by migraine. This affliction does not discriminate; we are strong people with marvelous achievements and fantastic careers in spite of the agony and fear we live with and illuminate here. We are amateur and professional writers, artists, and photographers; we are students, lawyers, nurses, laborers, social workers, sales reps, musicians, teachers; we are mothers, husbands, sisters, children, brothers, wives, and fathers; we are all ages and all people around the world.

Here, then, in our words and images, from our hearts and minds, in all its anguish and beauty... is life with migraine.

[1,2] Lifting the Burden, a collaborative global headache education campaign; www.l-t-b.org., Press release, March 15, 2007, and Introduction, statistic quoted from *The World Health Report 2001*, World Health Organization.

[3] *Conquering Daily Headache*, Alan M. Rapoport, MD, Fred T. Sheftell, MD, Stewart J. Tepper, MD, & Andrew M. Blumenfeld, MD, 2008, BC Decker Inc., Ontario, Canada.

[4] "The long drought: the dearth of public funding for headache research," RE Shapiro & PJ Goadsby, Cephalalgia, 2007; 27, 991-994, Blackwell Publishing Ltd.

[5] "Upside to Migraine Pain? The Case for Hyperthought," Michael Gaylor, 2007.

foreword

Migraine can be a very isolating disease. Even though Migraine is the 12th most disabling disorder in the United States, far too many people still think Migraines are "just bad headaches." Migraineurs are often thought to be complainers, slackers who don't want to work, or drug seekers. The stigma of such a misunderstood disease can make Migraineurs feel disconnected from family, friends, and co-workers.

Projects such as *Migraine Expressions* are rare, priceless, and sorely needed. They offer an intimate view of the impact of Migraine disease. The works of art in this book are deeply personal and revealing. They are both heart-wrenching and inspiring, filled with both terror and hope.

As you read and view the pages of this book, I know you'll be moved. I hope you'll be moved not to sympathy or pity, but to understanding and respect for those who live with Migraine disease.

Live well,
Teri Robert

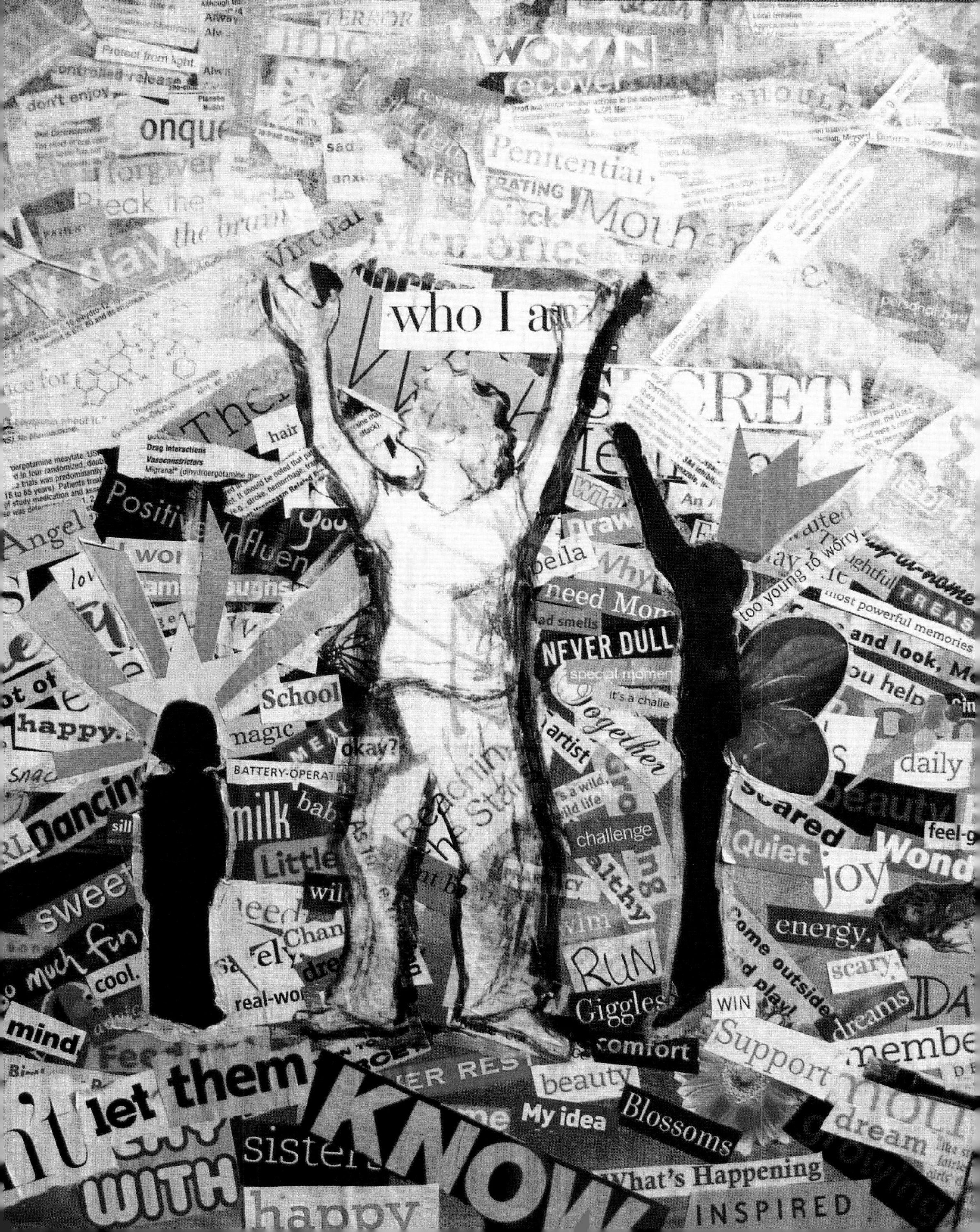

DON'T LET THEM KNOW ©2007 *A. Heather Davulcu,* Age 37, Yardley, Pennsylvania

A CREATIVE JOURNEY
through Life with *Migraine*

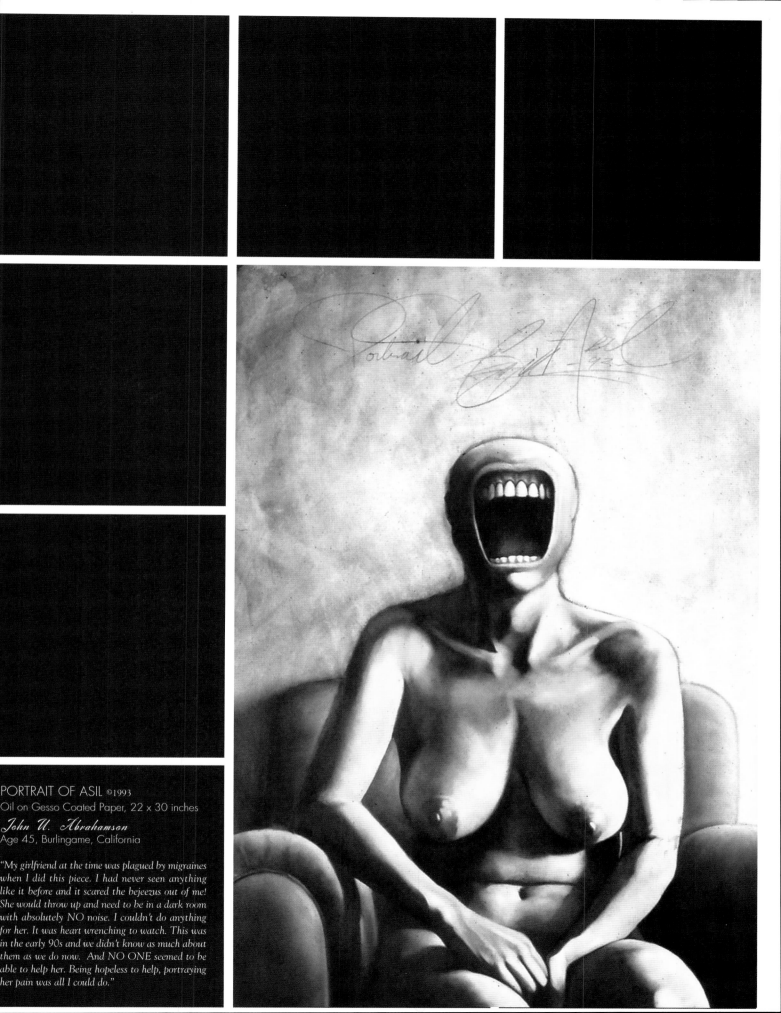

PORTRAIT OF ASIL ©1993
Oil on Gesso Coated Paper, 22 x 30 inches
John U. Abrahamson
Age 45, Burlingame, California

"My girlfriend at the time was plagued by migraines when I did this piece. I had never seen anything like it before and it scared the bejeezus out of me! She would throw up and need to be in a dark room with absolutely NO noise. I couldn't do anything for her. It was heart wrenching to watch. This was in the early 90s and we didn't know as much about them as we do now. And NO ONE seemed to be able to help her. Being hopeless to help, portraying her pain was all I could do."

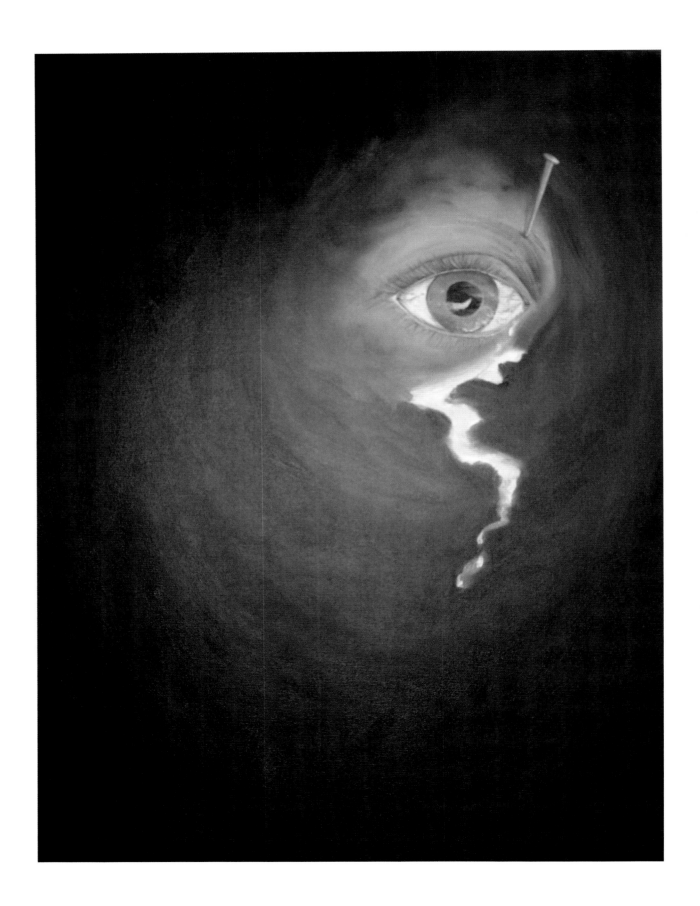

The Storm
©1995

Betsy Baxter Blondin
Age 54, Carlsbad, California

Oppression descends
And the storm's labor begins.
I witness the birth but deny the life.
Gray clouds pervade
and settle
in my brain.
I cannot focus through loose eyes
and dark distortions.
Lightning and thunder threaten.

The rain begins
and grows gradually stronger, falling harder,
pelting,
driving me into the black and lonely place
where blinding daggers of light
wait for me.

My stomach quivers with the shifting sky
and cannot be calmed.
Concentration agonizes,
movement is misery,
tears are torture.

I battle with obdurate denial,
fight the pain with paralysis.
Still it debilitates,
humiliates,
and mocks me.
Because even when the storm dies,
depression will cloud the sky.

Thus defeated again,
humbled,
I surrender to the storm,
acquiesce with the wind,
and envy the needle.

I lie down and allow the rain and tears to merge.

I am the storm.

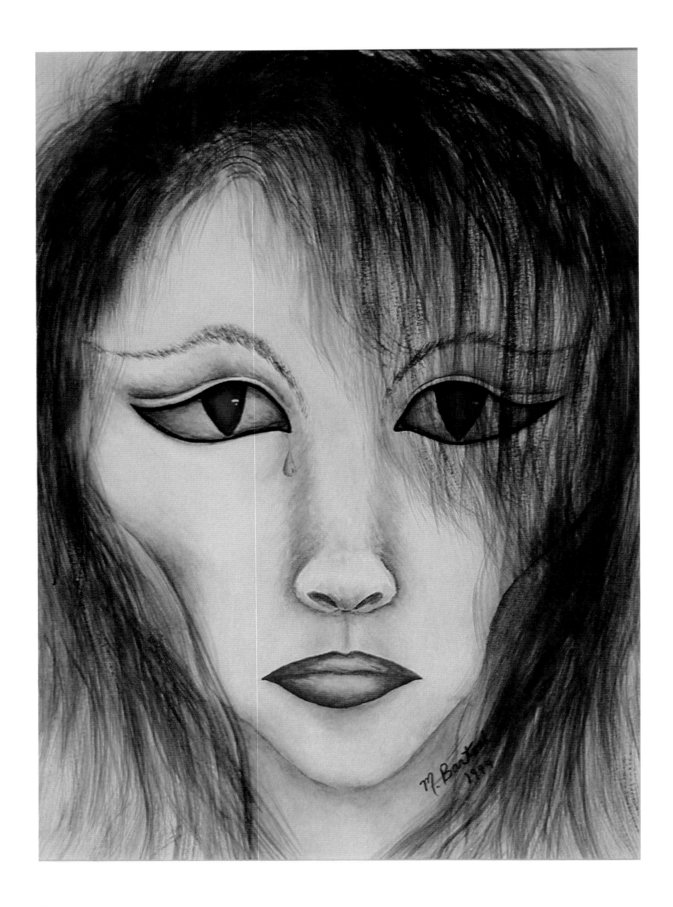

The Bright Sunny Sky
©2007

Melissa Bartosh
Age 40, Spring Valley, California

"Look out at the bright sunny sky and be happy to be alive." Did I hear this doctor correctly? Had he heard anything I said? How could he believe someone in severe pain every single day for over 10 years would want to enjoy the sunny sky, and be happy to be alive? I can't even bear to glance at the light, let alone enjoy it.

Be happy to be alive? Every morning I am greeted with pain from a skull that feels like it will explode, burning eyes that feel like they are bleeding tears, ears that feel like my brain is oozing out of them, a face that is half numb, vision that goes dark over and over, dizziness that makes the room spin and standing difficult, depression so big that life feels like hell on earth, and the whole day ahead of me to enjoy.

I go to bed feeling the same way. The next day I awake to more of the same with the added jackhammer pounding in my skull and with the ice pick digging into my eye. The newest visual effect is always a surprise. Spots, puzzle vision or maybe everything will just be a big hazy fog. Yet, this doctor is telling me to look out at the bright sunny sky and be happy to be alive. The sun is painful. It magnifies all these migraine symptoms. Shouldn't he know this? Why doesn't he know this?

I wish for death, but also want to live. I just can't live this way anymore. This is torture, not life. I came to this man seeking help, salvation from the pain, or at the very least, some small relief from it. Yet he offers nothing, other than to look at the bright light that blinds me and be grateful for my life.

I leave in utter amazement, in severe despair and complete hopelessness. I slide to the floor in this kind doctor's hallway and sob tears that only the walking dead can shed. This man has hammered another nail into my suicidal coffin. Somehow, I make it home in spite of the uncontrollable sobbing and gut-wrenching tears. Tomorrow I will once again awake to that bright sunny sky with a head that feels much too small for my brain, jackhammers pounding away, unable to even lift my head off the pillow. But, I am alive.

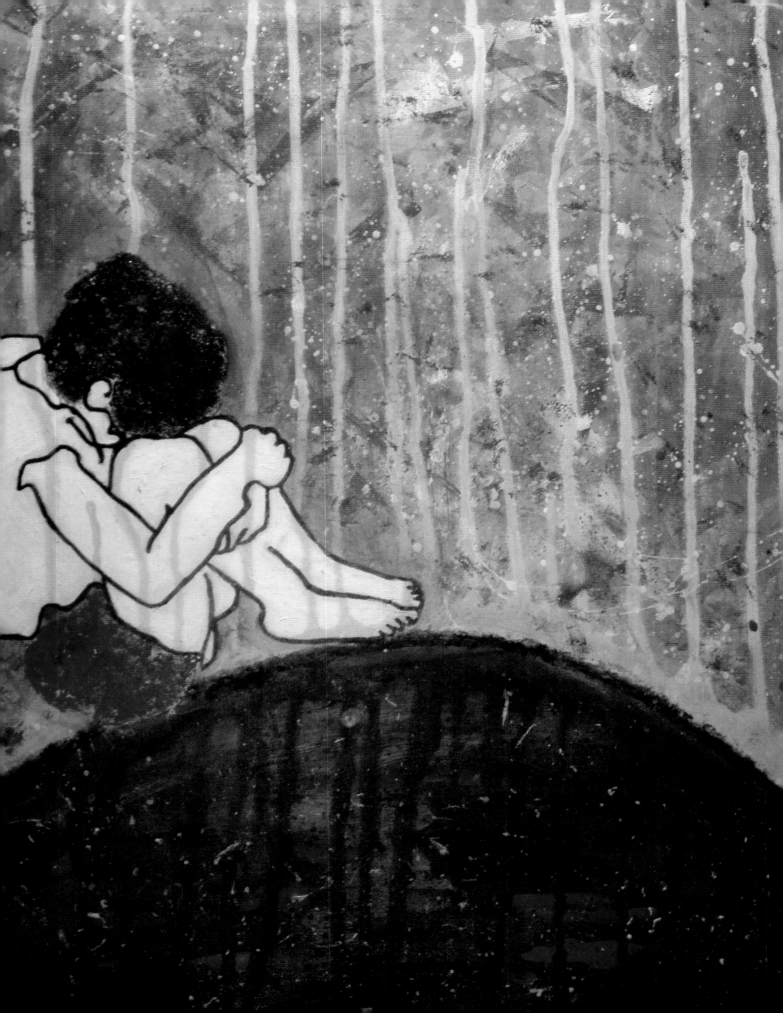

The Fish That Swim in My Head ©2007

Holly Harden, Age 40, Scandia, Minnesota

i call Abbott Northwestern. I want a CT scan. I want to see my brain on paper. I want analysis, diagnosis, reassurance that it's all there, all in working order. I will remain motionless in a large steel cylinder for as long as it takes. The words I want to hear? Your brain is healthy. Everything is in working order. You go, girl.

I am transferred to the proper desk, and I explain myself. The woman doesn't get it. Do you have a referral? she asks. I say no. Were you in an accident? Have you experienced bleeding? No, no bleeding, I tell her. But I do have an intense migraine every six or seven weeks. It always lasts three days. She is silent for a moment. She isn't sure what to say, and explains that their CT scan policy requires a patient referral from a licensed doctor.

Okay, I say. How about an electroencephalogram?

She seems annoyed. Are you epileptic? she asks. Normally, EEG's are done to monitor and facilitate treatment of epilepsy.

No, I say. I have never had a seizure, but I do have these fits now and then when I feel like my head is coming apart.

She is silent again. Then, what is your name?

I tell her. Listen, I say. What difference does it make whether I have a referral? If I am able to pay for it, why can't I have it done?

She is confused. I'm going to give you two names, she says. One is a headache specialist; the other is a psychiatrist. Perhaps they can help you.

Are you my referral? I ask.

She hangs up.

I don't need a shrink. If I have unresolved issues, I want to keep them. Imagine having nothing to work through. I'm curious, is all, about what's inside my head. Maybe I'm bored. Maybe, at 34, I want to learn something new about myself. My hands are restless. And, every six weeks or so, a school of small silver fish swim from the periphery across my retina. In the flash and shimmer of scales, I see a warning both frightening and familiar.

continued on page 24

The fish aren't large, reckless and writhing above the surface of the fluid in which they swim; they aren't pink-cheeked trout, spotted and sleek. They aren't the grotesque imposition of sturgeon. The fish in my head skitter and swarm, all together now, like neon tetras: magnetized, of one mind. They spring from the deep into the aqueous humor of my eyes, a fleeting school of grunion, a run of smelt. And when the lights appear, flashing and blue against the purple sky lining my forehead, I brace myself. These are lights of distress.

Within an hour, the fish have gone. I want them back. In their wake is a sudden darkness, a burst of black ink. The left side of my face has gone numb, except for the fault line, the thin stream of pain flowing from its gnarled source in my left shoulder, up my neck, arcing over my ear into the watery blue pool of my left eye. Its ending, where cornea meets air, is metallic and sharp. I am nauseated. My sinuses click with the static pressure, and I believe a creature gilled and green may find birth in my face.

I hear my blood in my ear: wish, wish, wish. My skin feels rubbery and damp; my nerves have turned their attention upward. I think about what is cool: a frozen washcloth; a bag of mixed vegetables; the newly forged head of an axe; wet sand. Then I think about the hot: steam; boiled cabbage; lava; branding irons; wax. I want it all — cool, then hot, then cool — against the softness called a temple. Not gently; this pain is beyond gentleness. It demands a worthy opponent. Pain negates pain. Let me rest my head in coals, then a bowl of frost. Call the Marquis.

No one knows why migraines happen. I have to eat. I can't do much about my hormones or my sex or my age, and I don't take drugs. I won't blame my serotonin levels or genetics, though the woman who gave birth to my mother, and my mother, both experience migraines regularly. So I'm thinking, give me the scan. Show me the breeding ground for my shimmering fish, and perhaps I'll find the answer for why, every month or two, I am forced to curl up in a corner with my eyes closed and fingers clenched and tread the waters of nausea and pain.

According to the medical establishment, the following "measures" may soften or eliminate the ache in my head: eat less meat and more fish; eat tofu; eat onions and garlic (they reduce clumping of platelets). Ingest magnesium, riboflavin, and fish oil. Cut down on wheat, chocolate, and aged cheese (and most of the foods I crave). Meditate. Check out a chiropractor. Apply finger pressure to the following places: the back of the hand where the bones of the thumb and index finger meet; the bridge of the nose; the hollow at the base of the skull; the base of the cheekbone; and the top of the webbed area between the big and second toes. Get acupunctured. Take caffeine and/or aspirin in regular, moderate amounts. Heat your body and cool your head. (Take a hot bath — add some dry mustard — with your head in a bucket of ice). Dip your finger in sesame oil, then salt and pepper, and shove it up your nose. I'm serious. And this is my favorite: avoid such lifestyle and environmental triggers as stress, sun, hunger, fatigue, sex, lights, loud noises, weather changes, and strong smells. (Or simply commit penacide, the suicide of the senses).

According to me, the following measures will effect, in some way, relief — if only momentary — from the pain of migraine: masturbate until your arm tingles and you think you feel a shark born of your head going after those blessed little fish. Chew, late at night, bark from the trees in your neighborhood, preferably oaks (easy to grip between your teeth) or willows (willow bark tea has been recommended for use in place of aspirin). But don't swallow; spit. Curse, loudly, as you spit. Sit in the middle of your living room in the lotus position and take deep, deep breaths. Blow out evenly, continuing until you pass out and tip over. The pain in your legs will, momentarily, ease the one in your head. Have your children, one at a time, as you lay curled in the fetal position, sit on your head and bounce, gently, humming "The Barney Song." If you have no children, ask a friend; or slide your head into a doorway, close the door as far as it goes, and prop it shut with bricks. Lie there until morning, or until someone knocks and says, "Oh, my God. Are you okay?" Don't speak; simply moan. Cover your face with a down pillow, and scream. Scream things that make no sense to anyone but you. Scream in other languages, in tongues, in rhyme. Scream Psalm 23 until your voice is hoarse and you're either laughing or weeping hot, salted tears. Find someone who loves you and beg him, plead with her, to do the very thing that needs to be done: find an axe, a machete, a drill. Use it. Peel back layers: hair, skin, bone. Dig until the fins appear, and cut the wild, writhing thing away.

As a child, in a Victoria, Texas, restaurant with my grandmother and two aunts, I ordered flounder from a large menu of items I didn't recognize. I knew flounder was fish, and I liked fish. The flounder came, eye and skin and tail, on a bed of rice. It stared back at me, and its gills were still as I nudged it with a fork. I ate little; it seemed forbidding and tasted fishy. I was trespassing. Where was the line drawn? Was I to eat it all, or to leave the fins or the skin out of some gesture of respect? And what about the eye? Where was the filet I had envisioned, pieces of which I'd dip lightly in butter? My selection was prescient: the next day, in the back seat of my grandmother's car, cruising up toward Arkansas, a small school of fish swam before my eyes, glinting and flicking

in a light whose source lay buried deep in the fissures of my brain. By the time we found a hotel that evening, the light had found my nerves, and my head throbbed like surf, pulsing with the coming in of a dark blue tide. Kill me now, I thought. I need water, I said. For three days, I drank only water, ate nothing at all, and prayed to Poseidon for forgiveness.

I am older now. I possess rabid hormones, menstruate, and do not have a steady relationship with my serotonin levels. I ingest caffeine, cheese, and cheap white wine on a regular basis, and am prone to the stress of being a "yes" person, a mother, and one of the self-appointed general managers of the universe; my ass is a trailer hitch for people in need. I take One-a-Day Plus Iron vitamins. I don't sleep enough. I straddle the barbed wire fence between the fields of random abstraction and concrete sequence. I am more than mildly interested, though on my own terms, in quantum physics. I am a practical, levelheaded woman. But still, in swells of pain, I creep outside at night and, spread-eagled on the lawn, call out to the sea god to quell, with his trident, the roiling within my head.

There is a dock on Lake Tahkodah in Northern Wisconsin where, if you lie still on your belly, hang your head over the edge, and immerse your hands in the clear water, the fish — sunfish, bluegill, perch, bass — will swim to you and kiss the tips of your fingers. If you reach for them, they deliquesce. You must be languid and still, and those fish, by the dozens, will love your forearms and the palms of your hands with the swish of tailfins and the fragile rippling of gills.

My next migraine is due, according to patterns of my own currents and riptides, in 11 days. I'm thinking, this time, of joining them — the fish — of slipping into the water, head first, through surface light, down through weeds and over muck, where things are cool and green. I have no gills. There are neither fins nor scales on my body. But I am streamlined; I have purpose. With my eyes wide open, my skin wetted and slick, I'll swim toward the deep where everything is remote and still. I'll become phosphorescent and grow a tail, and the fish in my head will swim out and along with me, a reasonable woman for whom the salt water of the open sea is the obvious cure for the ache of land legs and the stress of being human. ☙

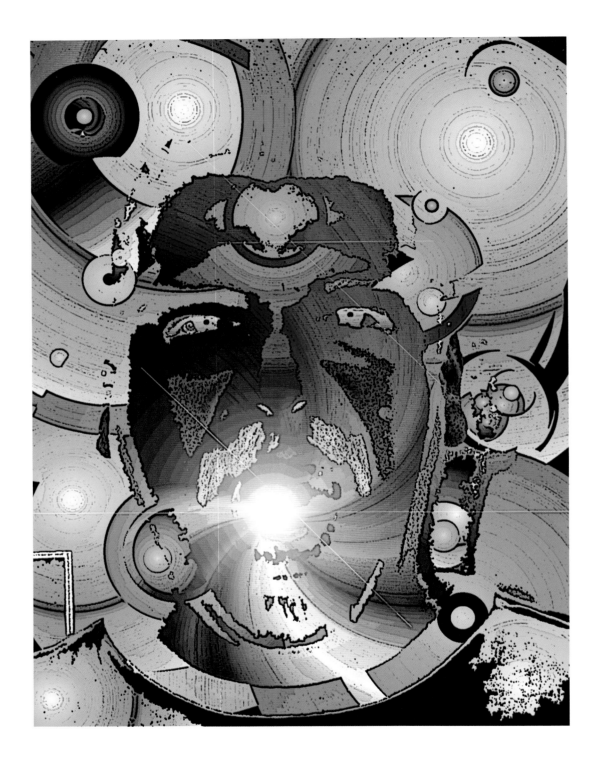

Migraine Band Practice

©2007

Michael Deasy Jr.
Age 44, Lacey, Washington

Fusion of burgundy seas laying out patterns
Twitching lights start to recede
Dangling sepulcher of crushing
Waste

Trilling light scorpions stick me with
Piercing piccolo noise
Fluttering above and around the night
Collapsing

Adding incense to flagellation, the
Marching band goes to work deep
In the abdominal walls, marchers denying
Even a horrid rest

Burying my face in quilts and shrouds
I take leave in an ocean of cotton
With spinning wheels of light and prisms dancing
Before my eyes

As I lie with the constricted thoughts and throbbing layers
Spending the last dimes of prayer possible
I quietly ask god to take me
She can't manage the mercy

TO ALL THOSE WITH MIGRAINES ©2007
I, too, share your brain cramps

Nikki Albert, Age 30, Leduc, Alberta, Canada

Yes, I share your brain cramps. And if you read 'craps' instead of 'cramps', we are on the same wavelength. I too have felt like my head was both exploding and contracting at the same time. I have also discovered that over time I know more of this disease than my doctor, neurologist and florist combined. From my decade of chronic migraines I have learned a great many things. I learned the hard way, via the school of hard knocks to the brain with a mallet. I have deeply contemplated all these things within my think box, aka, my bedroom. And I am here solely to impart my words of wisdom to you.

The pain is throbbing and feels like your brain is expanding beyond the compounds of your skull with the pulsing and the stabbing. A worm that threads its way through your brain or a piercing ache that spikes with movement. There are mild, moderate and acute migraines. And there are monster migraines, which can be the dreaded status migraine. Obviously pain is something to be avoided. It is, in fact, a blaring signal your body gives you so you can somehow stop it. Avoiding pain is the ultimate goal, unless you are a masochist.

Sometimes my hearing becomes muffled and at other times too sensitive. A customer may come into my work place and say their name is 'Fitzpatrick', but I may very well hear 'fuzzlebutt'. Sometimes, when someone is wearing a shirt with stripes (which simply should be banned) or standing in front of blinds, I am momentarily stunned by the pattern and cannot comprehend a word they speak. Occasionally, I lose my ability to understand simple sentences and when I speak I like to randomly substitute the word I meant for one that sounds similar but is utterly, utterly wrong. I may look at an object, such as a pen, and not be able to say what it is, except to refer to it as 'that thingy you write with'. I have learned to describe simple things with long descriptions so people will eventually get what I am referring to. I have also learned to edit my writing. My brain cannot tell the difference between p and d, c and o, 9 and p and likes to insert whichever it pleases. Likewise certain words are the same to me; site and sight, word and work. I may simply just forget how to spell. Or forget everything, like my address and my birthday.

I get the spectacular visual fireworks show, but the after show lacks in appeal. Still, no one else can claim they have seen raindrops of gold or translucent blue cascading though their field of vision. Although I find the double vision makes it hard to watch movies with subtitles.

You will not find me outside without a nice pair of sunglasses, my cheapest migraine preventative. I get tingling and numbness. The spastic twitches and trembling hands. Then there is the nausea, which I will just leave at that; The Nausea. I have experienced chest pains, vertigo and even outright fainting. This is the package combo that is a migraine. All the neurological fun.

Yes, I feel your pain and crazy neurological symptoms. However, how does one stop a migraine? Aside from the obvious; applying a heavy frying pan soundly to your head several times, until unconscious and repeat if needed.

First you must get rid of the triggers. The MSG, the nitrates, cheese and alcohol. And let's not forget caffeine and aspartame, which would be Diet Coke. I believe Diet Coke is more addictive than crack and substituting it with water was an unpleasant ordeal. And like any recovering addict I crave Diet Coke. It was a sacrifice that had to be made in order to find that elusive migraine-free day. You can try an elimination diet, where you start by eating nothing and slowly add things in, to find those sneaky food triggers. You may find that milk causes a migraine, whereas soy milk just causes an unpleasant taste in your mouth. If lack of sleep is a trigger, try sleeping. If it is hormones, try getting pregnant and staying that way, or, more dramatically, change your gender. If it is sunlight, become a vampire. If it is loud noises, wear ear muffs.

Next we come to supplements. If you like taking a fist full of pills three times a day, this is just the solution for you. I would suggest you begin with vitamin B's, magnesium and calcium. To start with. Add in some feverfew, some passion flower and valerian, with some chamomile for flavor. Just in case add a multivitamin. If you don't feel better, well at least you will feel full.

Most important of all is the blessed Abortive. A very expensive pill you take to abort a migraine. You take that pill, or stick that needle in your leg, or snort that spray and 'voila', like magic, the migraine is gone. However, don't take too many because then you get the dreaded Rebound Headache. If you get too many migraines a month, you then go for the Preventatives. There is an extensive list. You can even get combo platters. You can have Topamax with a side of Inderal. You can weigh out the side effects for the benefits. Weight gain, weight loss, and keep three sizes of clothes in your closet. Taste test a pill every few months until one satisfies you.

Lest I forget you might want to try yoga, acupuncture, massage therapy, chiropractic and physiotherapy. Drink a gallon of water a day and try standing on your head. Then there are always the headache cures that random people will suggest. Try them all. And then finally you may decide you want someone to stick BOTOX into your head, because if it does not work, at least you get the wrinkle- free scalp.

So you try all that and it does not work. Well you can use my frying pan method. That is some free advice, just for you, and a cheap treatment. Remember this list of preventatives is long. Try ACE Inhibitors, beta blockers, calcium channel blockers, antidepressants and anti-seizure meds. Try them twice, try them together. I find the side effects tend to be gas and migraines.

Still not satisfied? Well, I have a few things to say about migraines. Although your brain may very well feel like pudding and you may from time to time say pickle instead of potato, those who experience migraine with aura may experience less cognitive decline as they age. While this effect may be from the preventatives or from consuming mass amounts of aspirin in your lifetime, we will take this information with a grin anyway. There is also the myth that more intelligent people are prone to migraines. While it is a myth, you can still claim that your migraines are simply caused by your advanced intelligence and how you 'think' too hard.

Finally there is the benefit I like to call manic migraines. I cannot deny migraines give you a strong dose of the stupid. And I cannot deny that I can feel extremely lethargic before and after them. However, there are times when I feel quite the opposite to lethargic before a migraine. I get jittery and chatty. And, well, chatty is annoying, but still, I feel invigorated and full of mental energy. I can think clearly and quickly. Sudden insights and 'eureka' moments abound. Most importantly I get my most creative ideas when I have this buzz of neurological energy firing. Story ideas flow from me and even a mild to moderate migraine will not stop my creativity. I firmly believe anyone with chronic migraines should find a passionate hobby. Take up painting, writing, knitting or sky diving. Anything to help you express that confused intensity you hold inside. While a migraine may only be good for keeping my brain fresh, I find it is also great for inspiration, just not so great with the editing.

So just remember you too can reach the age of 80, intelligent, creative and sharp as a tack, with the most wrinkle-free scalp around. See, there is a bright side to everything. ꙮ

Song-less Morning
©2008

The house is quiet
The scent of banana touches the air
My heart sinks

I kiss your head.
I know you will make it through
You always do
I will wait as long as it takes…

For your smile, your song to return.

———

Wishing, Waiting
Once again we wait
For the waves to relinquish
The winds to wane
The tide to recede
So we can walk on the shore,
Wade in the water,
and wallow in treasure

———

It is deceiving.
You look peaceful, but we know you are fighting a great war.
And it hurts to know that no matter how many victories
we have on our side, the battles will continue.

———

Dear Mom,
Just so you know,
You never let me down. Your resilience, strength of heart and spirit,
your courage and perseverance inspire me.

©2008

Kelly Jo Blondin
Age 23
Montara, California

the monster lives inside of me
laying wait for that special moment
when he will rule
my every thought
my very being
He is my master
powerlessly I am pulled under
by the waves
of intense nausea
electrical cross-circuitry
a creeping skullcap of pain
probing my mind with sledgehammer cures
internal fireworks flash with great explosions of light
I can no longer see
this body is not my own
I belong to the tyrant
who savagely owns me
for today.
©2007

J.D. Blue
Plano, Texas

"Throughout my life I have had to stand by powerlessly watching loved-ones writhe in agony while their brain does the migraine short-circuit. My poetic expression gives voice to the victim bearing that unpredictable timer able to go off at any moment..."

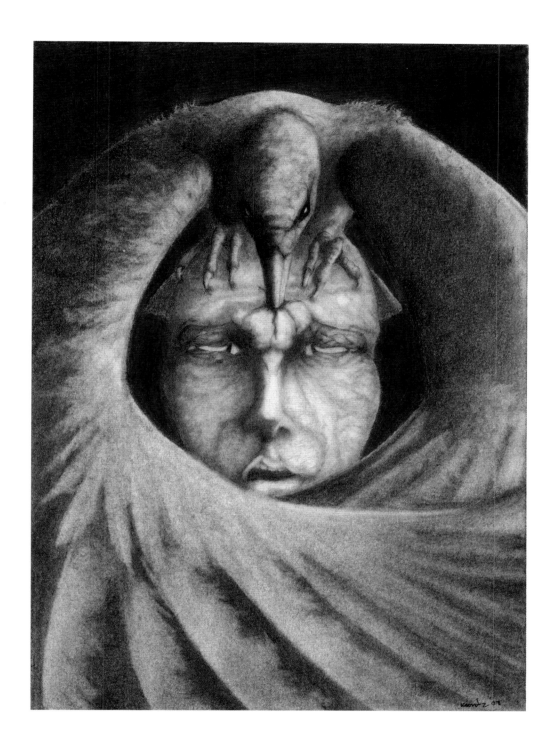

MIGRAINE ©2007 Colored Pencil & Graphite on Arches Sketch 8.5 by 11

Mark J. Koontz, Stanwood, Washington

"What makes them different from an ordinary headache?" My description,
"Like having a nail-studded corpse strapped to your head," didn't suffice, so I created a visual experience of migraine.

Cure
©2007

Erika Dreifus

It happened again this weekend,
This bright summer Sunday.
They'd invited their neighbors
For brunch on the screened-in porch.
But at six a.m. she rose.
It was coming.
The migraine.
By seven,
It had arrived.

She didn't open the drapes.
She simply sank back into bed.
Her husband tiptoed to the kitchen
To find more bottled water
And Advil.
Not that Advil helped much.
But why risk something stronger?
"Stronger" could be, had been, too strong, for her.
Cures really can cause more harm.

Then she fell asleep.
And while she slept
Her husband tiptoed again.
This time he settled at the computer
To cancel brunch.
And then he clicked on the television,
Keeping the volume low.
He only half-watched CBS Sunday Morning.
Listening, listening, just in case she called.

She woke.
Her head still rocked, punched, choked.
(Questioned later, she'd say:
"Like someone is driving a rusty nail behind my left eye.")
But in that moment she merely called for her husband.
"Maybe I'll try the new medicine," she said.
He found it.
The label said: "Use as directed."
But what, exactly, had the doctor directed?
With this brain, with this skull,
She could not recall.

Her husband called the pharmacy
(Not the doctor, not this summer Sunday).
He asked questions, and answered them.
"She took two Advil at six," he said.
"She weighs one hundred thirty pounds."
Then back he went to the kitchen
To slice a tiny pill in half so that this time,
Let's hope,
This cure would prove benign.

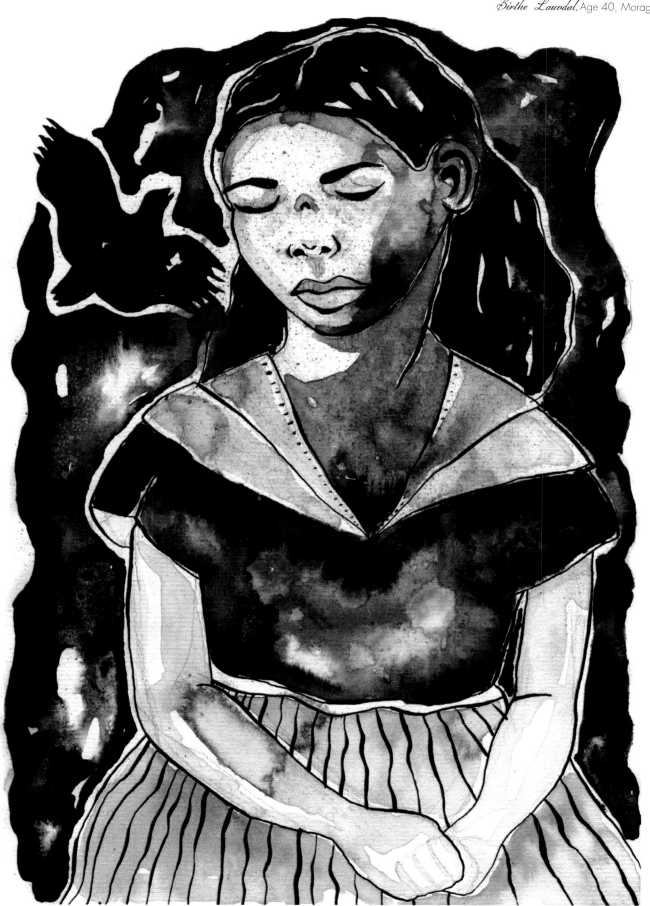

Riddle
©2005

David Morphet

It is an anvil ringing
with blow after blow.

It is bellows and coal
and the grip of tongs.

It is a diadem of steel
with torque and clasp.

It is the raw pith of a tree
stripped of its bark.

It is seen in an eye
which abhors light.

It is heard in the stab
of clocks in quiet rooms.

It is the teeth of a trap
clenched on bone.

It is an unhealed wound
to be borne alone.

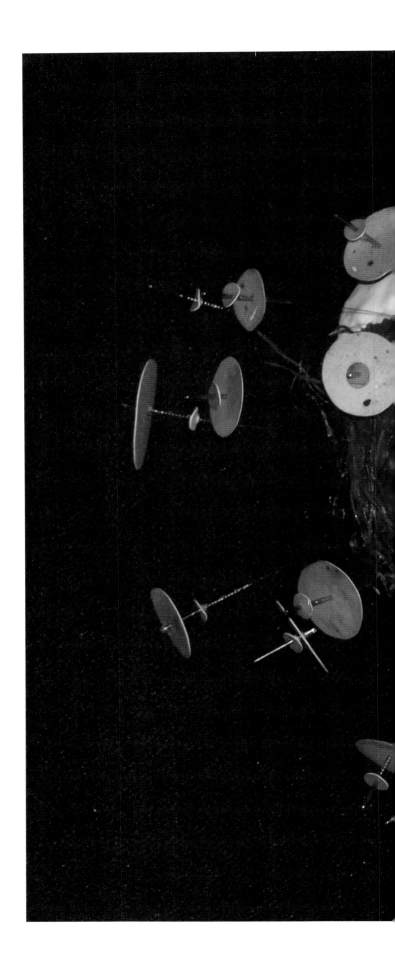

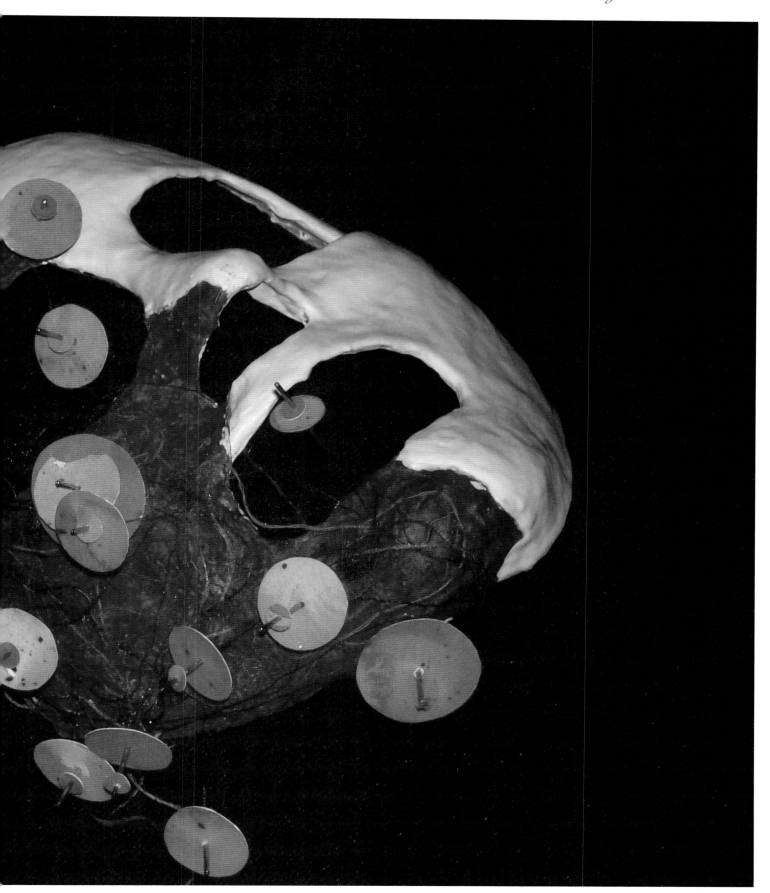

ME AND THE NIGHT VISITOR
A journey through a migraine ©1992

Pat Gallant, New York, New York

" If migraine patients have a common second and legitimate complaint besides their migraines, it is that they have not been listened to by physicians; looked at, investigated, drugged, charged, but not listened to." —Dr. Oliver Sacks

I know it before I awaken. As insidiously as it comes, the migraine finds its way into my dreams. The dreams are more vivid, usually nightmarish; though sometimes it is but an utterance of, "Oh no, a migraine is coming," and then a pallid recognition. Uneasy, I stir from sleep. There is a sense of ill-being: pain, weakness, lethargy and malaise. And with it comes the resignation that it must be endured.

My thoughts vary as I drift in and out of an anesthesia-like sleep. Sometimes the pain is so intense that I need someone to rub my head, my only relief. Then, I drift back into this quick, deep sleep, which is unusual for me, a light sleeper. I am certain my sleep cycle defies the norm on these occasions — entering REM sleep the minute my eyes close. I am pulled under against my will.

How can I describe it? Imagine having an intense headache, feeling groggy — as if on a sleeping pill — experiencing extreme weakness, all while riding on an ocean liner in a hurricane. This for a day, perhaps two, or more. Too sick for lights, phone, television, radio — only darkness. If I move, so intense is the sensation of seasickness that I feel dizzy, sick to my stomach, and my head swims. If I attempt to walk, I reel and feel faint. So, when the migraine is severe, I don't move, not even to go to the bathroom. I just lie still. It is during the worst of migraines that I fret as to what I would do if there were a fire and I had to get out. I am helpless. However, no matter how bad the migraine, I tell myself it will pass. The point is, they do go. I just have to get through it.

I have learned not to use migraines as an excuse. If I can't make the wedding or party, it is "the flu." Migraines just don't cut it. The thinking is, "Come on, if you wanted to, you could go. You're not trying. You're pampering yourself. It's all in your mind. It's psychological. You just need some fresh air. If I can function with a headache, so can you." The implication is always that one is giving in to the headache, that one is coddling oneself. With a high fever and the flu, no one wants to risk catching it, so no questions are asked, and no unwanted opinions are given.

People expect you to pop up after the migraine is gone, not realizing the exhaustion that comes after so many hours and days of pain. If one has just been in labor and delivered a baby, it is expected that one will need to rest. I had a 49-hour labor. It was nothing compared to a migraine. During labor I felt healthy, strong, and not even tired. The pains were very sharp, but between contractions, I was fine.

If I have a set of appointments, such as dental visits, I say up front that I get migraines and if I have one on the day of the appointment, I cannot come. I add, however, that I will pay. That's it. I'm tired of apologizing or explaining. I know it looks irresponsible to cancel. I've always been a conscientious person. It's hard for me to be viewed as irresponsible. This eliminates the judgments. Money talks. It costs, but it is only one of many costs of migraines. A higher price I must pay is being robbed of time with my son. I must also endure the frustrations of missed events, and of work piling up. I'm tired much of the time as a result of all the migraines. I'm always running, but I can't keep up.

I am fortunate to have a loving family that understands. They understand because they know me and they see the migraines. They see what a migraine is and what it does.

I wait for the migraine to go. It never fails to astound me when it does go — I am at last released. There is no thunderous applause, no standing ovations. But I know what I've weathered. I congratulate myself. Sometimes the migraine drops me off in the middle of the night, other times in the middle of the day. It has wreaked havoc with my circadian rhythm. If I am released at the wrong time, I must begin to slowly reset my inner clock. An abrupt time change will trigger another migraine. So, sometimes I find myself lost in time, out of sync with the world.

But the migraine has lifted. The air smells fresh again. Things feel good again. A sense of well-being replaces the sense of ill-being. I have yet to take the last step of the migraine, which is the requisite sleep, or the migraine returns. This last phase is a peaceful, quiet, and comfortable sleep. I can look forward to waking up renewed. But before I sleep, I take "my walk." My walk takes me to my son's room. I look at him, very glad to have him. I look out of the windows at the trees and flowers. I walk around the house and check everything. Everything is still in its place. Everything is still here. I touch things. The world is still on its axis. The house is still here. My people are still here. I am still here. Yes, I am still here... I thank God for all that. ⟫

"Sorry, not tonight dear, I have a headache," has been a long-standing "joke" of comics. But migraines are no joke. I hope "Me and the Night Visitor" will help illuminate a condition that has long been scoffed at and grossly underestimated. — Pat Gallant

"Me and the Night Visitor" was originally published in the National Headache Foundation Newsletter in 1992.

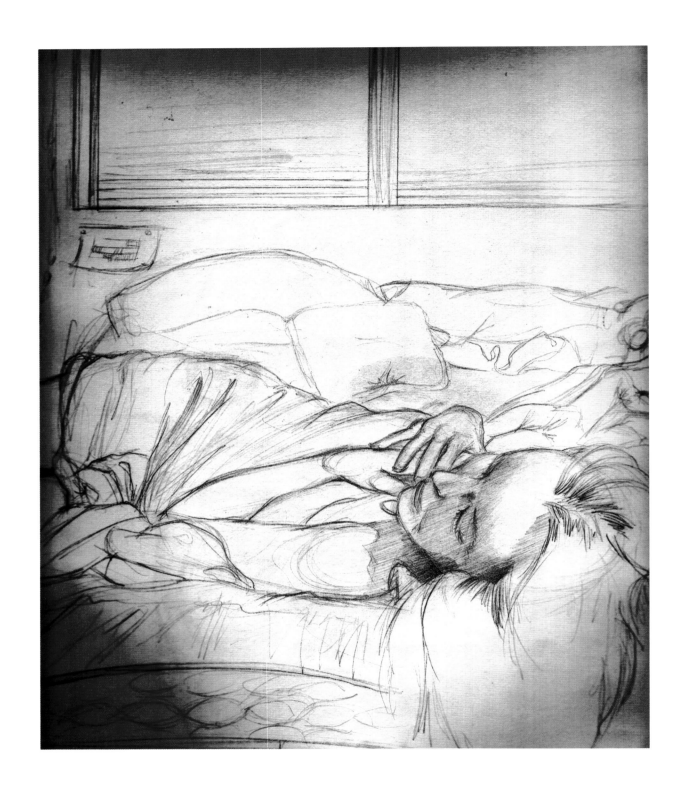

SLEEP ©2007
Nick Beery, Age 28

"My sister is a longtime migraine sufferer. Her misery always demanded attention from everyone who was intimately involved in her daily life.
Being close to someone who had to deal with the pain, nausea, and constant threat of an elusive affliction brought a profound influence on some of my most innate work."

The Egg Shell Dance

Nancy Bennett
© 2007
Vancouver Island, Canada

Older sister goes in first, making sure the coast is clear.
That IT has not returned.
We stand outside with hungry bellies and scratchy throats
careful not to clear them in case IT hears.
Time treads silent, daring not to tick
Should we kick up dust with our shoes? Dust covers the boredom but we dare not
as that sometimes "sounds like rumbling storm clouds" she has said, and IT
would know we were home.
She stands at the door, finger pursed to lips, socked feet and small breaths
motioning us with her eyes to go in.
We leave the noisy shoes that thud like anchors,
the jackets that might rustle
like breaking glass
outside.
One by one we move in slow
like soldiers in formation
we move as stealthily as we can, aware that IT has snipers
all around.
She and IT lay on the couch, under darkened curtains,
her eyes shielded with a dark wet cloth
and we know that now we must do the egg shell dance.
Careful not to tread too loud,
careful not to play or talk or whisper or breathe
or even ask for water for the dripping is like
the Chinese water torture, that's what she says
when she is here, not IT
and we can play outside, my sister signs, pointing us to go far, far off field
until IT has left the building
and we get OUR mother back.

Nancy Bennett does not have migraine but her mother did for her entire life, and her daughter, Amanda, who has artwork in this book, also lives with migraine.

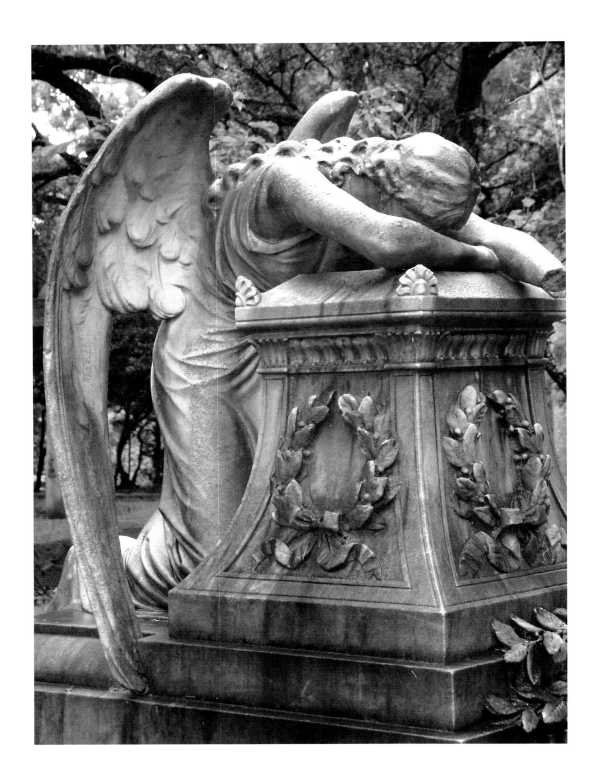

©2007 *Shana Pass,* Age 33, Houston, Texas

"Having suffered for years with migraines, this statue really spoke to me and I felt that others would see the message in the image."

Unexpected Sorority

©2007

Rachel Elaine Gordon
Age 41
Mount Kisco, New York

she also knows

the tendrils uncurl, drag you inside
pierce with light and sound and pain
throbbing, draws lifeblood to the core
it cannot explode
it tries

she also knows
the darkness
the silence
cool tile of bathroom floor
must not hit
must not drive that blessed cool inside your skull

she also knows
no wine
no cheese
no chocolate
no fava beans
(fava beans?)
pizza invites it in
feeds the talons of pain
no more, ever.

she also knows
Imitrex Maxalt Zomig
Migranal ergot NSAIDS
Demerol Fioricet
ACE inhibitors
calcium channel blockers
tricyclics MAOI inhibitors
SSRIs SSNRIs
all the rest

she also knows
'Have an aspirin'
'Get more sleep'
'Try these herbs'
'Eat better'
'Exercise more'
not our fault

she also knows
Lazy. Attention-seeking. Weak.
Selfish. Self-absorbed. Party-killer.
it takes strength to be so weak

she also knows
what it feels like to have this pain
to live with it always
to fight against it for life
for a life

to live with those tendrils always present
always possible
and to live
despite
and to live
compassion eclipsing agony
and to live
joy exists past the pain
and to live

she also knows.

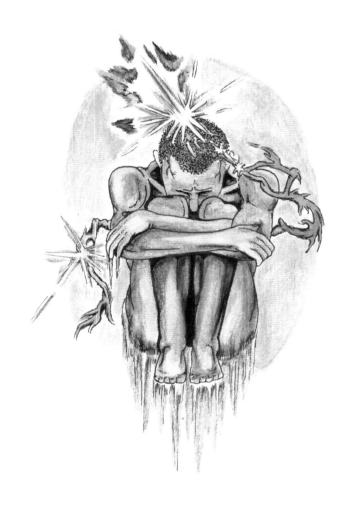

Pain
©2007

Kelly Maeser
Age 28
Omaha, Nebraska

I spend most of my life
In a pain-laden haze
In and out of days
I fumble and falter
Trying to cope
Giving up hope

I fade into the crowd
Lost and forgotten
Crying out loud
Through the smoke
That encases my brain
I look for hope to come through

A new dawn breaks
As I open my eyes
I can see the new day
Pain is forgotten
Anguish dissolved
My life renewed on the new dawn

Summer Cerebrum

©2006

Heather Nicaise
California

The dry Mojave dust swirls
around a tightened skull.
The Santa Ana winds

desiccated the earthworms
and left their bodies frozen
in the pavement mirages.

Lawn sprinklers pop
like mushrooms.
Snail shells crunch

underneath summer
sandals. Pain creeps
into sidewalk crevices.

Scalding cotton towels
turn into ice packs
beaded with sweat.

An endless late shift
conveyor belt of pills
delayed life.

I will not let my soul
be stolen or be stripped
by the lingering black hole.

I will find a way to mend
the shattered mirror
and find myself in its reflection.

"Even typically innocuous events can make migraine more severe. When the pain temporarily subsides, I force myself to pull all aspects of my life back together."

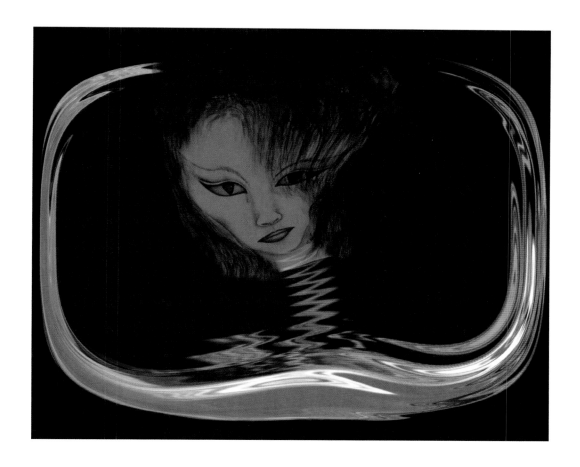

HEAD ON A SPRING ©2007

Kay L. Williams Houck, Age 62, Pen Argyl, Pennsylvania

Kay Houck is the mother of Melissa Bartosh, whose work also appears in this book, and they both live with migraine.

THE GEOGRAPHY OF PAIN © 2007

Daniel Hudon, Age 43, Somerville, Massachusetts

When I think of the Canary Islands, I think of driving down a deserted road with my fellow astronomy grad students until we found the restaurant where I had one of the juiciest steaks of my life. I think of relaxing over a cerveza and tapas, particularly tapas pulpo (octopus), after the workshops with a French student from Marseille. I think of precipitous views from winding cliff-hugging roads. And I think of driving with Gustavo and Diane around Teide, the volcano tall enough to create its own weather, and through the surreal lava formations of its moonscape basin while suffering a piercing headache — a migraine.

The sun's light faded on the panorama and I felt like a broom handle had been jabbed into my eye. I remember thinking, "Maybe this migraine will help me remember the scenery." As we weaved down the darkened roads, catching glimpses of tropical plants in the headlights, Gustavo, who was driving, said, "I think we're on another planet." It was true. Each turn brought on some ghostly, barely visible spectacle, but I couldn't concentrate anymore. I began to wish we would just arrive already so I could lie down and be relieved of consciousness, of wakefulness, of even the small task of taking in scenery.

One of my greatest fears in travel, besides forgetting my passport or the plane going down, is that a migraine will strike when I am on the road, far from the comfort of a cool, dark room, an ice pack and a soft bed. It has happened to me in Guatemala, in Laos, and in a Himalayan village in northern India, where I spent several afternoons drinking chai and chatting with a sadhu named Baba in the crisp mountain air while steam from the hot sulfur pools warmed our backs. I was having a relaxed day, I wrote in my journal, until I got clobbered by this migraine. It has shot a hole through my head, my left eye is a vortex of pain.

I went to visit Baba and he gave me some balm to rub into my temples. After a few moments I told him, "My temples are burning."

"It is the pain coming out," Baba replied.

It wasn't, of course, because the migraine lasted for a while longer, but the balm did provide a temporary distraction.

On the road or at home, I have battled migraines for more than 20 years, though I remember a few severe headaches from my childhood. Once, when I was about eight years old, I got to stay up past my bedtime to watch a hockey game on television and I was determined to take advantage of the situation… I remember squinting through the pain. When I was about 12, I missed playing in a football game at a family reunion because I felt like the side of my face had caved in and I had to lie down.

They started in earnest when I was studying for final exams in my third year of university. I was an astrophysics major and that year I had a heavy load of astronomy, physics, and math courses. I bought some classical music tapes in the hopes that they would help me stay at my desk longer. They did, and I've been a dedicated fan of classical music ever since, but they couldn't prevent my migraines, who became a frequent afternoon guest. In solitary confinement in my room, I had a strange existence where, after the migraine hit, I

would take some pain killers and study as long as I could stand the pain, nap for an hour or two and go back to studying without anyone knowing what I had endured, both in my head and in my head.

I remember a bit of doggerel I wrote around that time: "Can you hear the war going in my head? My brain lies bleeding, nearly dead." But I've tried not to let them interfere with my life and tried to live my life despite them. For years, I didn't want to talk or complain about them because I knew the stories about others who suffered much more severe migraines: a complete inability to function, temporary blindness, or days of pain.

Still, my journal kept the score:
— like my head was too heavy and began imploding from its own weight;
— like a visor of pain that came down from the top of my head;
— my skull feels like it's 10 sizes too small;
— when I finally crawled out from under the shadow of pain…

One day's entry begins, My headache has left me, as if that single sentence can summarize hours of throbbing pain. Another entry sums up the frustration: I've had a headache all afternoon. I'm probably allergic to something like blue jeans or air.

I never had the classic warnings — the aura or flashing lights — just a dull pain that grew, like the sound of an approaching jet, until it couldn't be ignored. In Canada, you can get aspirin with codeine over the counter, known as a "222," and I would take a pair of them. I slept or took another pair an hour or two later and usually, after a few hours I would be pain-free again. Usually. But I didn't want to take pills for any minor pain in my head on the chance that it might erupt into a migraine and often delayed taking them, with predictable consequences.

My family doctor wasn't much help. Despite my regular onset pattern and the fact that the pain was localized behind my left eye, he said they were just tension headaches and to keep taking the 222's. "I don't feel stressed," I told him. I slept normally and as far as I knew, wasn't irritable. In retrospect, I think the 222's worked about half of the time and for my two or three migraines per month, I spent a lot of time trying to sleep them off.

Among the classical cassettes that I bought was one of Gregorian chant and I used to put that on when I lay down, an arm thrown over the side of my caved-in face. It was like sinking into my own funeral and I entertained a range of morbid, depressing thoughts about never being rid of the pain. But the chant soothed until sleep would at last relieve me. If the migraine wasn't gone when I awoke, I felt ripped off, that the time invested in my sacrifice was inadequate.

Sometimes I listened to a cassette by a Canadian band called Courage of Lassie. They played soft, wistful pop arrangements and I still remember the opening lines from the album, Temptation to Exist:

"You walk in the room, and that's when you know

She's by the window, as though she isn't home."

These were companion songs for a life put on hold, a comfort for the loneliness of pain.

Sometimes I would come home from work with a migraine and sleep through the entire evening. Waking around 11 p.m. or midnight, stunned at the storm now past, I would get up, go into the living room and salvage a few hours of reading — well into the middle of the night — before I was tired enough to go to bed and sleep until morning. In fact, under the tent of lamplight, these became cherished hours where I felt lucky to be alive and reveled in the quiet feeling that the whole world was sleeping but I was temporarily excused.

I have tried a variety of remedies, including cold compresses and hot showers, soaking my feet to get all the blood out of my head, neck massages, which rarely helped, and foot massages (courtesy of girlfriends), which sometimes did. I have tried hot cups of tea and hot soup because I remember each of them worked once and so I keep giving them another chance. I have tried deep breathing exercises and relaxation techniques, which have perhaps taken the edge off the pain, but more importantly, feel proactive, so I keep trying them. (As for yoga, downward dog, alas, gives me a headache.) I have even tried masturbating, which was at least a temporary distraction from the pain and the only time I never had a twinge of Catholic guilt.

Often, I picture the migraine as dozens of thin, sharp sticks (the sort used in the Pick up Sticks game) hoisting up my brain. When the pain reliever starts to work, if it does, I imagine the sticks being removed one by one and my brain settling down again. In the throes of an attack, I wish I could open up my skull and grab the whole bunch of sticks at once.

Sometimes I've imagined a surrealist self-portrait of a large head of cauliflower with a fork stuck into it. The title: Still Life with Headache.

Sometimes, I remind myself, It's only pain. Or, more dramatically, This too shall pass. Or, I think of what my father would say: "Well, I guess we should amputate."

Meanwhile, I have seen other doctors, had an MRI, and tried various prescription preventatives — calcium channel blockers and beta blockers — with the only notable result being the side effect of depression.

After a particularly bad episode, I bought a book about different types of headaches and slowly began to make connections to food (I had already regulated my sleeping patterns and meal times). This has been an endless, tedious process made more difficult by the fact my sensitivities have changed and foods that used to be harmless are now on my DO NOT EAT list. Composing the list has taken years of vigilance and sometimes thousands of miles. In Thailand, where they always cook with fresh ingredients and the food is delicious all over the country, I discovered peanuts were a migraine trigger for me. Goodbye peanut sauce, peanut butter, green peas and snow peas. I miss you. In Turkey, also a great culinary nation, I added green peppers to the list. I miss them too, together with red peppers. I miss cooking with onions and I miss popping garden-fresh cherry tomatoes into my mouth and exploding them.

I haven't been able to keep track of which red wines are high in tannins so until then, they are no longer worth the risk. I miss a nice glass of port wine after holiday dinners. I used to create wonderful concoctions out of leftovers, until I connected them with migraines, due to a chemical that builds up while the cooked food sits in the refrigerator. Now I cook just the right amount. But I miss a slice of cold pizza for breakfast. I miss ham or roast beef sandwiches for lunch. I miss olives and olive oil, though the former still tempts me on occasion. (Here, I wince because I was never an olive fan until I met a terrific woman who loved olives. She said she trained herself to like them because "The people who like them like them very much." I trained myself to like them — and to love them. Now, not only did I not get the girl, but I don't get the olives either.)

I miss eating everything on my plate, the way I was raised.

The 222's stopped working long ago and now I'm onto triptans like Imitrex. I try to catch the pain before the sticks get raised again, with reasonable success. And I take fewer risks. I used to be optimistic that some of my food sensitivities were only temporary and so I would try the food again months later hoping for the best. Now I know the result and don't even try anymore. I used to experiment with fancy cooking sauces. Now, I eat simply, with only fresh ingredients.

The vigilance is paying off and I think I've turned a corner. Until I identified soy milk and olive oil as triggers a year ago (formerly part of my daily diet and neither of which used to be a problem), my frequency had shot up to two or three per week, nearly driving me crazy, but now I'm back to my old average of two or three per month, and it's decreasing. When I go a week without one, I get a strange sense of euphoria, like I'm finding my way out of the labyrinth.

After all these years of battle, I still don't know how much my migraines have affected me, how they have shaped my outlook on life, my capacity for suffering and empathy of others, or whether, less likely, they have merely been annoying. I do know that I'm grateful that we can't remember the sensation of pain once it has past, only the fact of it. And I've learned not to take anything for granted, particularly a relaxing afternoon or evening. At times, it has been like driving down the curved Canary Island roads at dusk, not knowing what's coming next. I just keep hoping there's a cerveza and some tapas at the end. ❧

Rebekah Jorgensen, Age 25, St. Paul, Minnesota

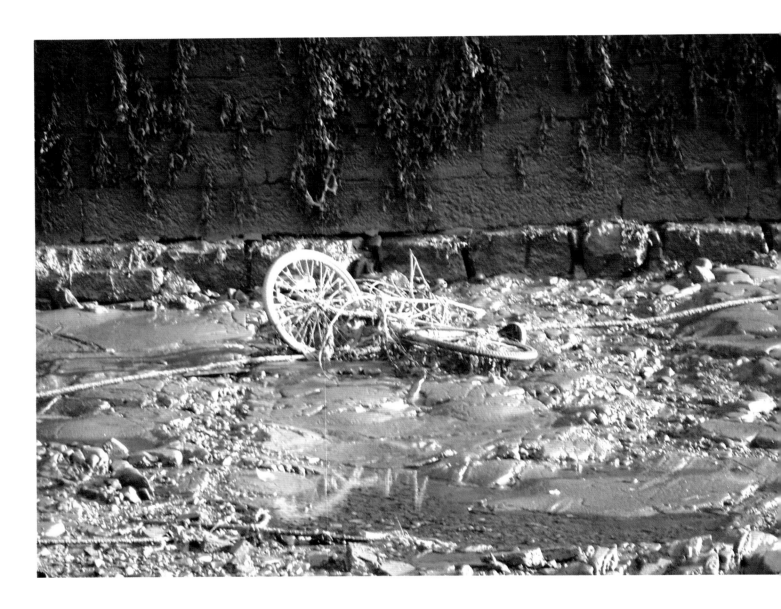

Gray ©1999

fog
rain
nails
smoke
chains
clouds
old age
pad lock
handcuffs
eggshells
beer cans
machinery
metal safe
cold steel
bird's nest
mousetrap
barbed wire
office carpet
business suits
cigarette smoke
chain-link fence
the mind

Rebekah Jorgensen
Age 25, St. Paul, Minnesota

*"The poem, written as part of a school assignment
shortly after my first migraine, and the photo, taken
on a more recent vacation to Dublin, are not so much
the migraine itself as the aftermath, the worn-out
exhaustion left behind, and a portrayal of the link
between depression and migraines."*

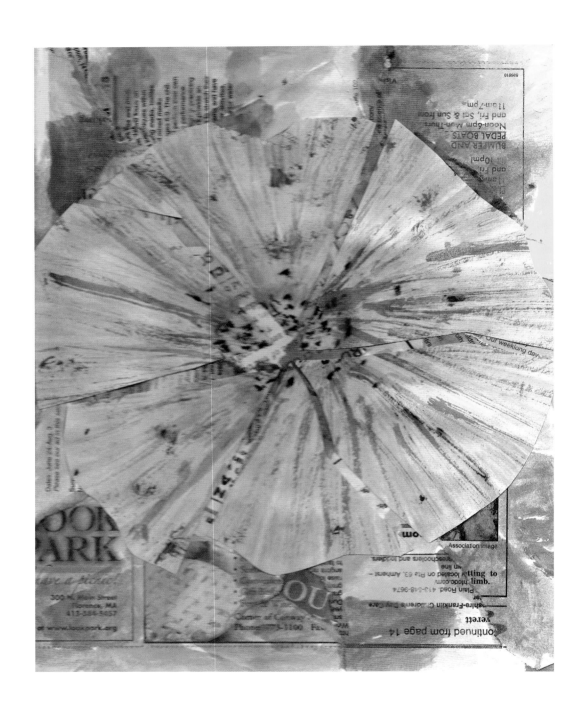

©2007 *Katie Sapp*, Age 23, Dracut, Massachusetts

"Every head has its own headache." —Arab Proverb

Ballet
©2007

Katie Sapp
Age 23
Dracut, Massachusetts

it's a dance, in half time. time step-step-step-half step-step-step step. i can't always see with these eyes, but i walk with pointed toes pointed north, magnetic north, tip toeing to places my eyes cannot see. rub my sweaty palms down the thighs of these faded jeans and tap my fingers -two-three-four and keep a beat to keep from losing it. repeat what you know — two-three-four... you are a girl -two-three-four... you live here -two-three-four... it is a new year. dancing june bugs in january mean my eyes are on siesta til i can blink them all away which is never. tango onto the bed and tangle into the sheets and cover my head underneath unwashed jersey sheets that smell like me but who am i again? i am a girl -two-three-four. you live here -two-three-four. keep it together -two-three-four. anxious eyes try to catch every moving spot they know don't belong. winter rainbows paint my walls electric red and black and green, and when i blink into a close, i can spin onto the ground, never once hitting the floor. round and round and round and —shhhhh.

CANOE COVE ©2005

Jackie Taylor, Age 24, Medicine Hat, Alberta, Canada

"This painting is inspired by the beach of the same name in Prince Edward Island, Canada. It is one of my favorite places to visit and unwind. It is a beach I enjoy going to when I can, but it is also a place that I am able to close my eyes and visualize when I am in too much pain to think of anything else."

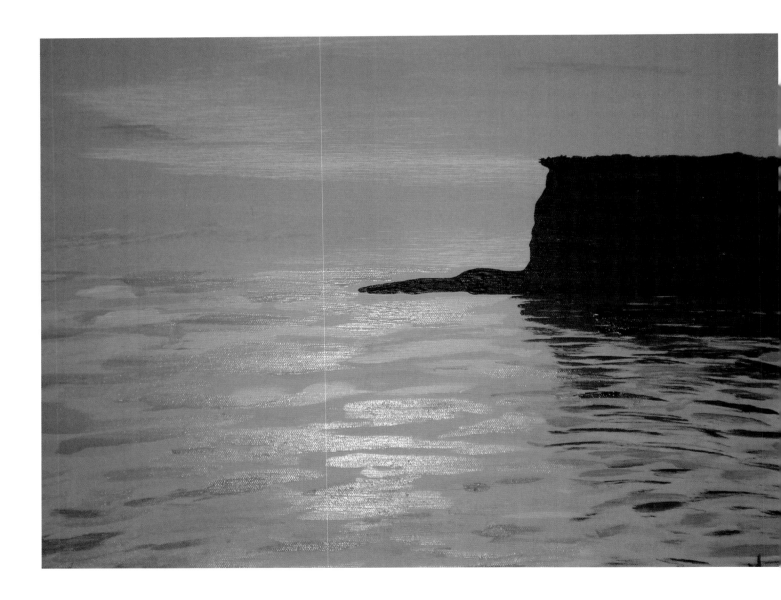

Ceaseless tides in and out,
I wait, wishing for the treasure they hide.
Only a glimpse this time,
Then footprints swept away.

The surf suffocates, surrounds,
I wait, wondering
Where did she go?
When will she return?
What can I do?
Nothing.

Powerless against the ocean's omnipotence
I linger by the shore,
Knowing
Only time will reveal
The treasure I call Mom.
©2008

Stacy Ann Blondin
Age 23
Boston, Massachusetts

RACCOONS ©2000
Melissa Bartosh, Age 40, Spring Valley, California

"These three raccoons were orphans I raised while also rehabilitating other sick, injured and orphaned raccoons. Knowing I was needed by these critters helped me get through an extremely difficult time in my life. The pain and depression I felt during this time was severe, which made living life quite unbearable. But I had these raccoons looking to me to help them survive, and that helped me persevere. Their little masked faces with their cute hands gave me hope and helped me believe that there was something more to life than pain."

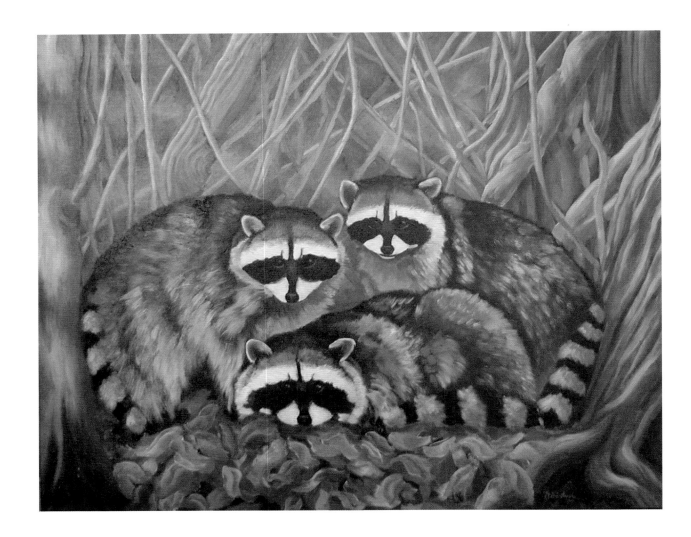

Migraines, Cats and Me

©2007

Harriet Cooper
Toronto, Ontario, Canada

I wake up and, like a bather testing the temperature of the water, I check the level of pain in my head.

On good days, I bound out of bed. Well, I bound as much as I can with a fat cat perched on my chest yelling for breakfast. On medium days, when a gentle current of pain eddies around in my head, I rise slowly, willing each step not to swell the surf into tidal waves.

On bad days, like today, I lie back in bed and wonder what sins I committed in past lives to be visited with such punishment in this one. I swallow, willing myself not to be sick. Although I'll feel better if I throw up, the thought makes me gag. Besides, it's been 12 hours since I ate and my stomach is empty. Instead, I concentrate on breathing, counting each breath to give my mind something to think about other than pain and nausea.

Unfortunately, cats don't understand the concept of migraine. All they know is they're hungry and the giver of all food is falling down on her job.

"Five more minutes," I whisper and pull the covers over my head.

By now a second cat has joined the caterwauling. The left side of my head pulses with each yowl. I scrunch my eyes tighter; it doesn't help. Soon one of my cats will dig under the covers to bite me.

I cautiously turn on my side and raise my body, the way I was taught in yoga – slowly and carefully so as not to jolt any part of me. I ease my legs over the edge of the mattress and rest. The cats have bounded off the bed and are swishing their tails against my legs to urge me to hurry.

But when you have a migraine, the word "hurry" doesn't exist.

Several deep breaths later, I'm ready to stand up. My feet find purchase on the floor and I inch myself off the bed. I straighten my back one vertebra at a time until I'm halfway between Cro-Magnon and Homo sapiens. For now, a round-shouldered stoop is as upright as I'm going to get.

I half-shuffle, half-slide into the next room to feed the felines. Once their dishes are full, they ignore me.

I continue shambling into the kitchen and grab my migraine medication. Third day in a row. Not good. This week has been particularly stormy and, for me, changes in barometric pressure cause migraines. Even though the meteorologist hadn't called for rain, my head told me differently. I've learned to listen to my head. It's seldom wrong.

I lurch back to bed. Luckily today isn't a teaching day so I have the luxury of sleeping through the worst of the pain. I pull the covers over me and castigate myself for having had too much coffee and chocolate the day before. While these substances, unlike red wine and colas, don't usually trigger migraines for me, I can never be sure.

Within 20 minutes the medication kicks in and the top layer of pain dissipates. As I drift off, a furry bundle plops himself against my hip, another plants herself on my legs. With their stomachs full, they've come to offer comfort and warmth. Either that, or they're hoping when I wake up again I'll have forgotten I already fed them.

I don't care. Right now, which is the only time that counts when you have a migraine, they're a loving antidote to pain.

Tomorrow, I tell myself, will be a better day. The cats purr their agreement. ❧

HOPE FROM DESPERATION ©2007

Kerrie Smyres, Age 31, Seattle, Washington

temples in a locked-down vise. Circus elephant balancing on one foot, spread across my forehead and nose. Head throbbing like Fred Flintstone's big toe after he's dropped a bowling ball on it. Ears as sensitive as cheese grater-bitten fingers. Nausea that could only be induced by deep sea fishing. Skin and scalp as tender as the chicken breast I had for dinner.

This is how I feel a couple days each week. The rest of the time, I still have a headache, it just isn't that bad. Yet I think I've had success in treating the migraines that I've had for nearly 20 years. I still have pain, mental fogginess, nausea, an outrageously sensitive nose and many other largely unknown symptoms of migraine. They just don't intrude on my life in the same way as they once did.

I have had migraines all my life and chronic daily headaches beginning when I was about 14. I sought treatment when I was a teenager, but doctor after doctor dismissed my headaches. Although it is now clear that I have migraine, my symptoms don't fit the classic model of migraine that was the migraine benchmark in the mid-90s.

With no diagnosis and desperate for relief, I sought a solution on my own. TMJ and sinus surgeries were the most dramatic attempts, but there were also allergy shots, a mouth guard, massage, exercise, acupuncture, an energy healer, and lots of Advil and caffeine.

Only after my headaches became so severe that they woke me in the night every single night, did I stumble upon a doctor who paid attention. Although he couldn't relieve the pain, he gave me immense comfort by acknowledging my suffering as real.

Diagnosis in hand, I thought finding a treatment would be easy. I was a great patient. I gobbled up every medication or supplement I was given.

Nine preventives, five abortives, IV therapy, daily injections of DHE… Nothing worked. Not one bit.

Yet I still believed that I would be migraine-free one day. I looked for my miracle as if I were window shopping. I looked through the glass at all the possibilities. Every time I started to walk through the door, thinking I'd found what would provide relief, the metal grate slammed down at my feet. I stuck my fingers through the grate, but could never reach far enough to touch what I needed.

Desperate for relief, I had an occipital nerve stimulator implanted. An experimental treatment with little indication of its potential effectiveness, it felt like my only hope. For almost three years, it kept me from practicing yoga, running, kayaking, riding horses and any of the many other activities that might cause the wires to move.

Within two weeks after the surgery, I knew the relief wasn't significant. I thought it helped, but couldn't — and still can't — quantify how much. Learning that my last hope didn't make me even close to headache-free was devastating.

My heart-wrenching grief was indescribable. In more than a year of clinical depression following the surgery, I had to face that there was nothing left to reach for. That my miracle treatment does not exist.

The only hope for my emotional relief (other than the lovely cocktail of antidepressants I'm still taking) was to accept that a pain-killing prince will never save me. The perfect treatment for my migraines and chronic daily headache

may come in my lifetime. I just haven't put my life on hold waiting for its arrival.

It may seem like I've given up. It's hard to explain that I feel acceptance, not resignation. Hope isn't about expecting to find a magic bullet. It's understanding that I can have a full and joyous life despite my illness.

In *The Anatomy of Hope*, Dr. Jerome Groopman defines hope as "the elevating feeling we experience when we see — in the mind's eye — a path to a better future. Hope acknowledges the significant obstacles and deep pitfalls along that path. True hope has no room for delusion."

A better future does not require living without disease. Yes, people often overcome illness or are able to live without pain. But not everyone does. A better future can also be learning to live joyously even with debility.

A few years ago I didn't understand the distinction. The time I spent denying the reality of my illness kept me going, for which I am thankful. I am even more grateful that my current version of hope is rooted in reality. A reality that means I spend more days than I want in bed, but that I'm not in perpetual emotional agony.

Believing that I can live a happy, successful life even with migraine and chronic daily headache requires constant maintenance. I am forever reminding myself that I could fight and get nowhere, or accept migraine's constant presence in my life and lessen its impact. Still, finding hope feels at times as nebulous as finding a migraine treatment.

One of my strategies was to find a visual symbol of hope. Something I can see every day to be reminded of my strength. The ever-changing clouds of Seattle became just that. Their colors, density and position in the sky take dramatic shifts throughout each day. Unless the sky is a uniform gray, there's always something to admire.

Like the clouds, sometimes my pain is light; other times it is unbearable and accompanied by a host of other symptoms. The changes occur from day to day, hour to hour. Even on the darkest days, I catch glimpses of blue sky.

Plenty of my days are perfectly described by the dense, dark gray overhead. I've become grateful for the variations in my headache clouds. They give me hope that headaches won't destroy my joy. Even if I have a headache every day of the rest of my life, the subtle changes within a day make me appreciate every moment I have.

My other daily reminder is a quote from Winston Churchill that was inside the lid of a bottle of Honest Tea: "If you're going through hell, keep going." Although I hate to admit that I got inspiration from food, this has become my mantra.

My life is the constant game of trying to balance caring for myself without becoming paranoid about my triggers. To take care of myself within the boundaries of illness, but not hide under the covers.

I live more deliberately and try to take advantage of every opportunity I have. Maybe I can't commit to an eight-week writing class or take an African dance class. I can take pleasure in a walk around the block or a great cup of coffee. I am fully engaged in the everyday as well as the bigger things I get to do. I have to rest, stay out of the sun and be constantly vigilant of my triggers, but I am more aware of the joys of traveling and seeing my favorite band play.

It's a cliché, but my life is richer because of my illness. The times I've been incensed by reading that in an essay are innumerable. I've become one of those people against my will. I'm not saying that all you have to do is change your attitude or that it's easy. Getting here was a long, excruciating process. I wouldn't wish the agony upon anyone, except that I want everyone with migraine or chronic illness to share in the beauty that lies on the other side. ❧

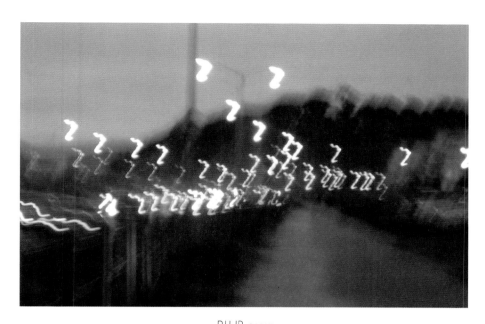

BLUR ©2007

"Sudden pulses of light creating a center of confusion and how some migraines feel when they linger beyond the point of understanding."

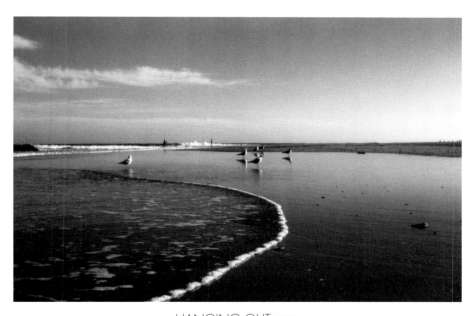

HANGING OUT ©2007

"At last a sense of relief and natural connection is reflected in this image of bird life by the sea."

Ladislao (Lollie) Ortiz, San Francisco, California

The Usual

©2006

Teresa Cantilli Ramos
Age 46
Garden City South, New York

I hate to be a complainer,
because lord knows I could complain every day,
and that gets irritating and annoying
and who wants to talk about it really
If you ask I will just say —
the usual

Yes, I see you looking at me with concern
I look pale, tired, frightful even
If you ask I will just say —
the usual

Sometimes you can tell that I have a horrible migraine
It shows in my face, my eyes, the way I carry my head
If you ask I will just say —
the usual

I certainly appreciate the question,
but sometimes just talking is a hardship
I will just do what I need to the best I can
If you ask I will just say —
the usual

There are times that I will feel worse,
and times I will feel better,
If you ask I will just say —
the usual

*Poems in this book by Teresa were originally published by
Teri Robert in the Putting Our Heads Together Poetry Contest on
MyMigraineConnection.com.*

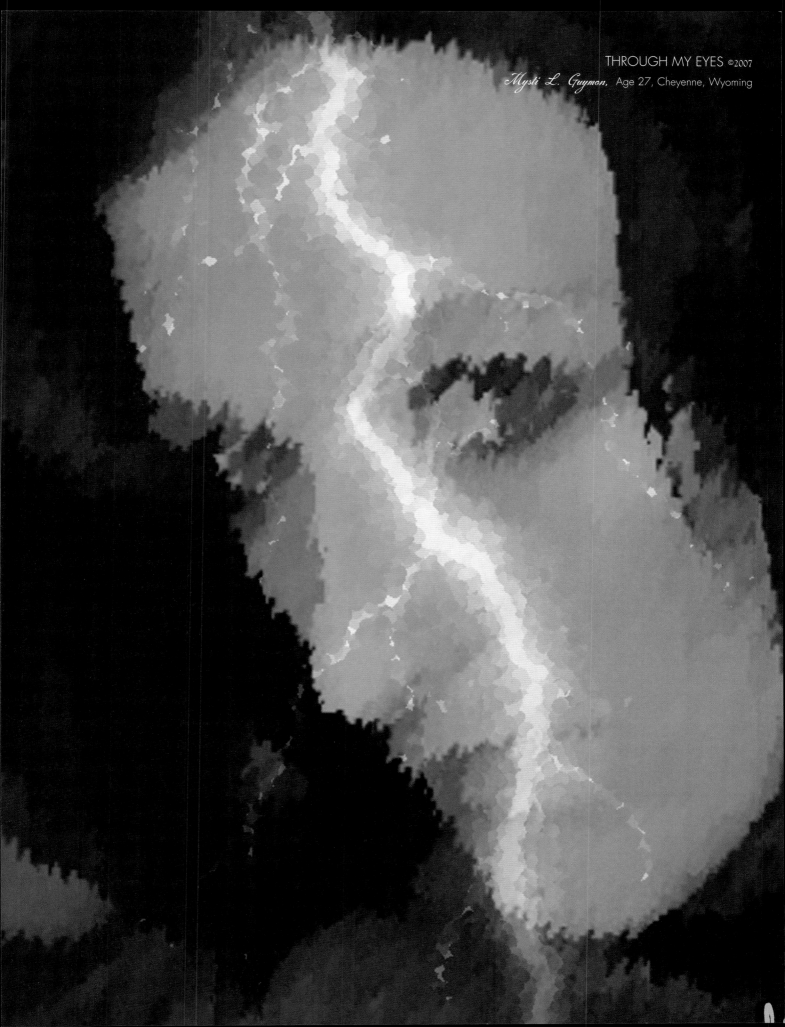

ON MY HEAD ©2003, Oil on Linen
Linda Horsley, Age 58, Seattle, Washington

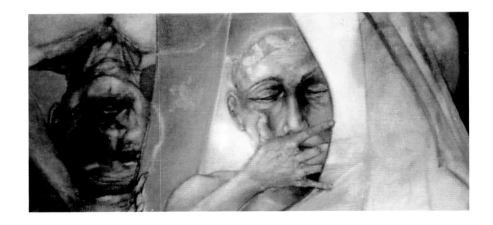

Embraced
©2007

Linda Horsley
Age 58
Seattle, Washington

My hands reach to hold the piled moments
of linear time which fills this space I am in.

Leaving this atmosphere of folly
and spitting pain,
head high and pulled back by
ancient crusty collectors of bones,
I choose to dive toward the scream,
turning away from blindness,
and put a fist in the sleeper's mouth.

I have done everything
but stand on my head
to escape the pounding inside me.

Now I have only to embrace the light,
grabbing onto the sharp horizontal line,
and pulling the memory of being lit
toward me without suffering.

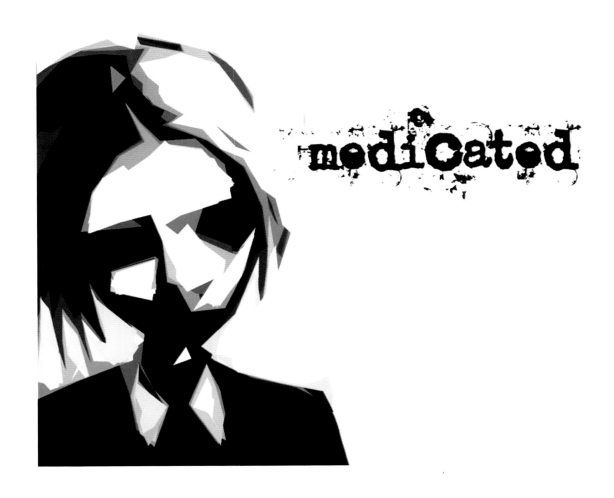

MEDICATED ©2007

Tim Dankanich, Age 32, Philadelphia, Pennsylvania

"Health care has become a drug-dealing business. Money is in the treatment, not the cure."

From pinprick small to vise grip tight
my headache roams to travel light.
Not far to go inside my head;
better off enduring root canal instead.
No doctor can explain why
my off-kilter serotonin levels endure;
I don't cry as much as in the beginning.
Little brown vials decorate,
suggesting an unexpected education
as those child-proof safety caps
are uneasily opened, revealing nothing at the surface
but vivid or pastel colors,
masking muscle quivering side effects
and other chemically induced changes.
Almost one year past the point of origin —
chronic pain and meteor shower sparklers,
invisible to others but for the inevitable
grimace, wincing as it tightens
from frayed loose ends to one taut knot.
What I've got is a daily reminder
of nothing more than illusion.

sumatriptan soliloquy
©1998

Lori Shapiro
Age 45
Marlton, New Jersey

My-Graine: My Pain
©2007

Shamoyia Gardiner
Age 15
Miami, Florida

The storm crashes around me
Tidal waves of pain consuming my sanity
My peace, the serenity
It's gone

Thunder rolls, I cover my ears
I feel it resonate within me, myself
The sound owns me, and then to prove its strength,
It tosses me aside with a mighty roar
A roar of laughter
A roar of pain
A roar of ownership
A roar of power

I crawl into a cave, clinging to my shred of protection
I cover my ears, screw my eyes tightly shut
I hope against hope that the storm will pass
And then
Lightning strikes
My vision swims with purples, pinks, and blues
My eyelids are, for the moment, transparent
I catch an unwanted glimpse of throbbing blood vessels
And realize
That the pain only gets worse
With every passing second in this storm
This horrible torrent of anguish
Is intensified by a new onslaught
Of hurt
Of light
Of sound
Of unfairness

I cry
Ibuprofen just doesn't do against this
I can't fight it
I must rest
So I slip into unconsciousness
And let my eyes shut
And let my mind calm
And let the storm pass

And silence and darkness cradle me

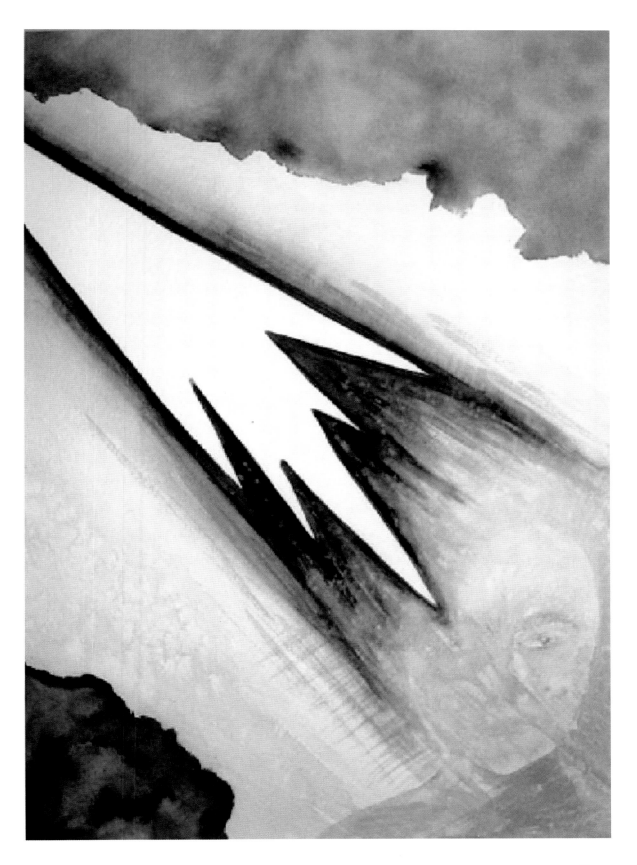

MIGRAINES IN RETROSPECT ©2007

Mary Litchfield Tuel, Vashon, Washington

a therapist once leaned toward me and asked, "What would you give back to your father if you could?" I laughed. "His headaches!"

Possibly not the answer the therapist was looking for, but certainly the answer that came to mind. All the time I was growing up, I remember my dad passed out on the couch, lying in the dark. He took tons of painkillers, starting with aspirin and moving up the chain of efficacy. I remember seeing him standing at the kitchen counter one day, swilling down codeine cough medicine, trying to get a little relief.

I know from my own experience that codeine isn't that great a relief for migraine pain. Never worked for me, anyway.

My first migraine hit when I was about 27. I was in a difficult relationship, and I blamed the headaches on tension and stress. I'm sure the tension and stress did not help, but after I left the relationship, the headaches stayed with me and came more frequently.

I would have, on average, four or five headaches a month. First came the aura. I never saw lights or had any other visual disturbances, unless the thing that happened occasionally when everything I looked at became like a grainy photograph and slithered around qualifies. I don't know. When I asked a doctor about it, he looked at me funny and said he'd never heard of that.

I would begin to feel tired; oh so tired. My eyes began to water. My nose began to run. A little tiny pain began in my temple, the precursor of what was to come. Light became unbearable. The pain increased, the nausea moved in. I retreated to my darkened bedroom with cold rags and a bucket, and waited, waited, waited for the pain to pass. It built up for several hours, usually was its most intense for about four to six hours, then began to taper off for another four to six hours before I began to feel like I was almost myself again. Then the next day I'd get the other headache, on the other side of my head. Whee.

It took a long time to realize I was having migraines. I thought that if you didn't see things, it wasn't a migraine. Every time I wanted to believe that this time the headache wouldn't develop; the pain and nausea wouldn't happen. Denial in the face of undeniable reality.

For years the headaches ruled my life. I was afraid to apply for a job, because I didn't think I could show up reliably. I missed days of my life, lying in that bedroom in the dark. Once a migraine started, I knew my goose was cooked for the duration, and I dropped everything and headed for home, and the bedroom.

Somewhere in there I realized that the migraines were connected to hormonal swings in my body. There were times of the month that I could rely on having a headache. The only times I had any relief were during pregnancy and nursing, before my periods returned. Looking back, it's a wonder I didn't have more children just to get those months off.

I gave up eating dairy and lost weight but did not lose the headaches as the naturopath had promised. I used Excedrin, washed down with coffee, and that made the pain at least bearable. I discovered ibuprofen dulled the pain, but it caused intense pain in my gut if I took it more than once a day, so I only used it when I had to. As time went on I took Excedrin and ibuprofen together, again washed down with coffee.

A prescription drug called Midrin helped — I was lucky. It doesn't work for a lot of people with migraines. Ergot and Imitrex made me incredibly sick before making me a little better. I was already throwing up; it didn't seem worthwhile to take drugs that added pain. I took Vicodin and other class 2 narcotics — not effective, and made me feel stupid besides. Threw the rascals out.

I tried everything anyone suggested: feverfew, magnesium, chiropractic adjustments, massage, long walks, icy cold water on my head followed by hot water followed by icy cold water, ice packs applied to the back of the neck and to the temples; head bands, acupressure, acupuncture, fasting, prayer, and diets — lots of different diets.

When I finally got up the nerve to get a real full-ime job, the first day I went to work I got a migraine. After working there for a couple of years, my supervisor said to me one day, "Can't you do something about these headaches?"

All I could do was look at her. Do something? You mean there is something I haven't tried? Something that works?

That is one of the most frustrating things about having migraines. People who don't have migraines really don't get it that you are sick and you're doing everything you can. You're not looking for sympathy (though that would be nice); you're not loafing; you're not trying to get out of anything. You're missing days of your own life and your children's lives; you're missing work; you're missing out on your relationships with spouses, partners, friends, and family. You're missing whole chunks of your life, and people who don't understand think you're just lazy or neurotic; and if you're really having headaches, it's your own fault somehow. They also don't understand that while the headache is the main symptom of the disease, the whole body is involved. Your head might feel like it's exploding, but your whole body feels like crap. There are also migraine attacks without headache pain.

Occasionally I'd try to get medical help. One nurse-practitioner told me that because I only had four migraines a month, I didn't qualify for a new drug. My situation wasn't serious enough. Obviously this person had never had a migraine.

My husband, unfortunately, has had migraines. That experience, coupled with his kind and generous nature, made him incredibly understanding and supportive. I am so blessed in him. I know that many people with migraine do not have the understanding of their partners and that relationships end over it.

I finally hit menopause a year or two back, and the headaches began to come less frequently. I had hoped and dreamed that this might happen, because the headaches were so clearly tied to my hormonal cycles. I have not had a migraine now for months. Knock on wood.

When I talk about migraines now, it's as if it is a story about someone else. It's a story about a woman who didn't know when she woke up in the morning if she'd be able to do everything she hoped to do that day: cook meals, pick up the kids, sing some songs, take a walk. Hold down a job. I always knew that whatever I was doing I might have to stop abruptly and retreat to my drugs and darkness.

I'm older now, and I feel like I was cheated out of a lot of my life. I try not to be resentful about it or dwell on it, but I can't help it. Oh well. I got a lot done in spite of my migraines, and maybe they made me a little more compassionate and understanding about other people's chronic conditions. I'd like to think something good came of it, but I don't know. It seems like a lot of pain for no good reason. I certainly connect with other people who have migraines. I don't miss having regular migraines, and I live forever with the knowledge that I could wake up with one again tomorrow. ᴑ

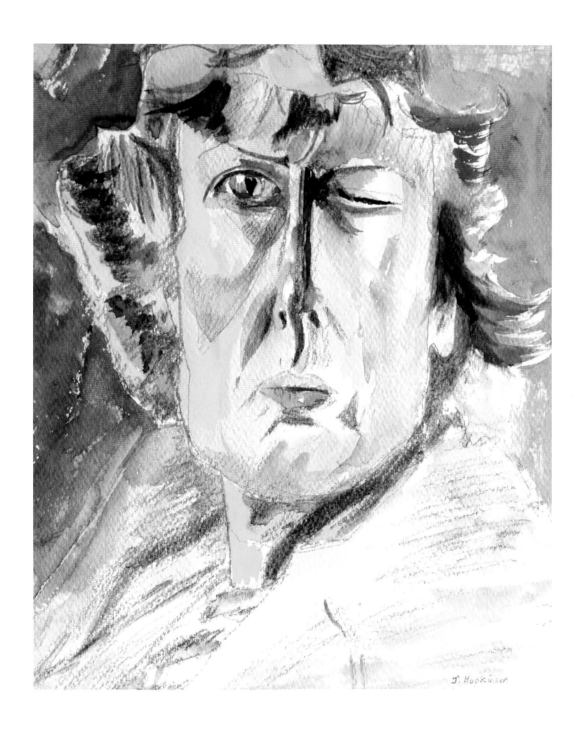

PORTRAIT OF A MIGRAINE ©1995

Jenny Hopkinson, Palo Alto, California

"I woke with piercing head pain. The rising sun stabbed my eyes. But my funny reflection in the mirror made me smile, so I recorded this migraine in watercolors."

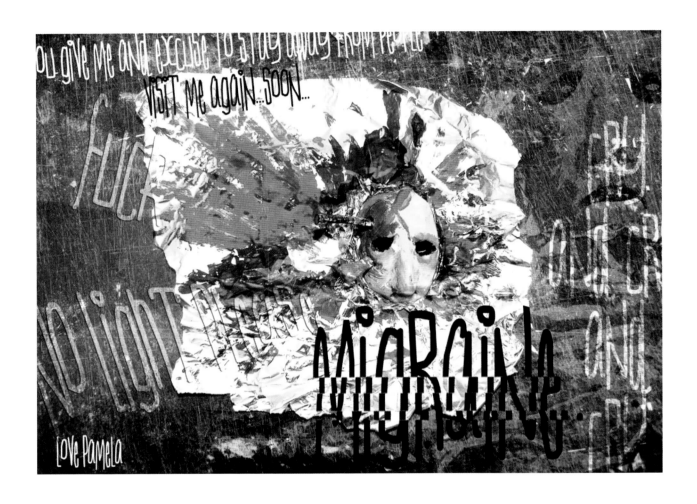

Incorrect Enclave of Imagined Salvation

©2007

Elizabeth Weiss McGolerick
Maryland

The middle-aged woman and her
elderly mother sit with their backs to me
but they might as well be on my lap,
on the floor at my feet, begging attention
like the puppy I have yet to purchase.

She's that singer! squawks the daughter.
Who? crows the mother bird.
The one who just had a baby and now
she's pregnant again! says exasperated daughter.
It goes and goes. Hard of hearing

and hard of speaking two rows
in front of me in the waiting room.
The second irony connected to this
head doctor of mine: macaws let loose
to cackle about nothing of importance

but attention-getting for the sheer decibels
of voice. The first irony: I come to him
to heal the trouble with what's upstairs
but he puts me on hold, victim
to an ear-raping concerto.

An upbeat tempo to peal through
my ear, reverberate on tiny drum,
and make my reason for seeing him
flood back full-force. There is a ringing
in my ears, doctor, from your on-hold music

heavy on the violins, the mother
hens in your holding area, the way
you look at me as though I frighten your
stability. I saw your pharmaceutical rep
walk to your back office with Ho-Hos

and Twinkies in a plastic supermarket bag.
Handle me with sugar-coated kindness.
Give me a parting gift. Make me like you
so I'll believe that you might actually care.

The Mask

©2004

Melissa Bartosh
Age 40
Spring Valley, California

Don't be fooled by the face you see. For it is a mask that hides the pain, such incomprehensible pain. Shrieks of agony ring out, eyes bleed. Tears make an ocean of bloody pain and sadness that just won't stop. There is no end to the drugs, side effects, lost life and lost dreams.

I could be; I could do so much, but I am all alone behind the mask that imprisons me. No one knows what is behind the mask. No one knows the secrets of this prison. No one really wants to know anyway. They don't know what to say. They don't know what to do. They try to help, but it's fruitless. It's all been tried before.

The pain and sadness continue. People turn away. Some even run. And some don't believe me. That is the worst.

The pain continues every day. No one wants to hear about it. I see it in their glazed-over eyes and I hear it in their silence. The mask is what makes them happy. Why have everyone in misery?

They have no idea of the misery behind the mask. None whatsoever. It imprisons me in a tortuous hell from which I cannot escape. No key exists to free me. I wish so much for the day I can burn the mask.

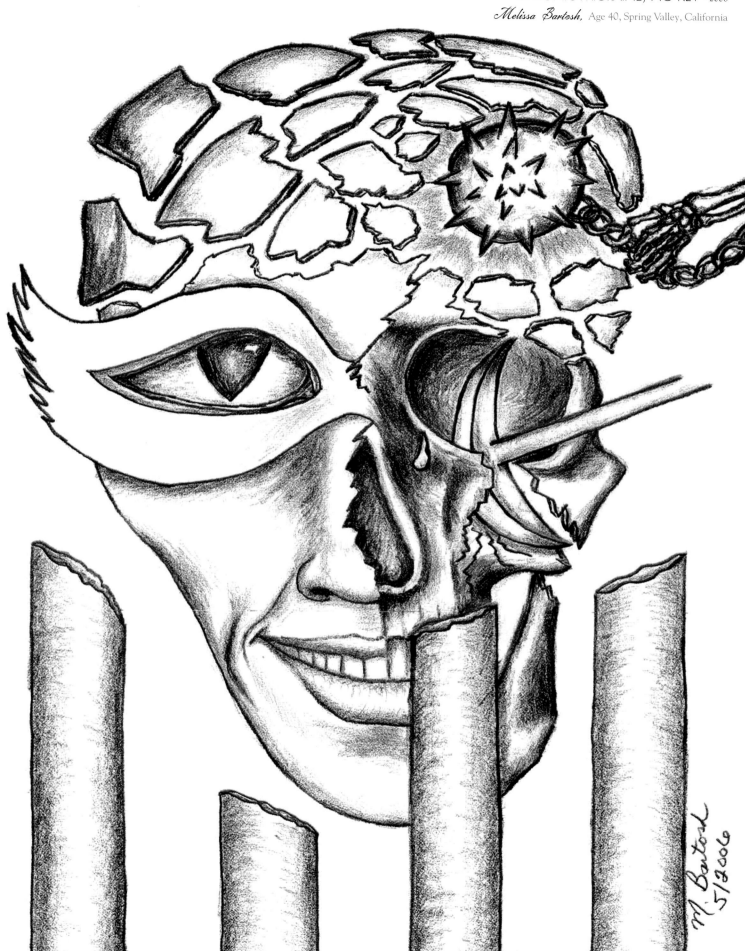

a comment on
migraines and subtitles
©2004

Kayt Hoch
Age 46
Seattle, Washington

I didn't see
the alien ship
last night because
I had a migraine
and was lying on
the couch under a
green towel with
my sunglasses on,

or maybe it was
that the aliens
didn't notice me
wearing sunglasses
in the house
because they landed
on the couch looking
for a green towel,

or maybe the
aliens knocked
on the door
looking for a
green couch
because they had
a migraine,
but I was busy folding

towels and didn't
recognize them because
they were wearing
sunglasses – I'm not
entirely certain – I know
I didn't see the ship
land, but they
were definitely here

because I woke up on
the couch with my sunglasses
on and heard them
speaking French
somewhere by my bookcase,
and even if I didn't
see them land, they must
have come from somewhere.

*First published in HazMat Review, Vol. 6 Issue 2
Winter/Spring 2004*

Reprinted in Ha! Magazine *Vol.1 No. 1, Spring 2004*

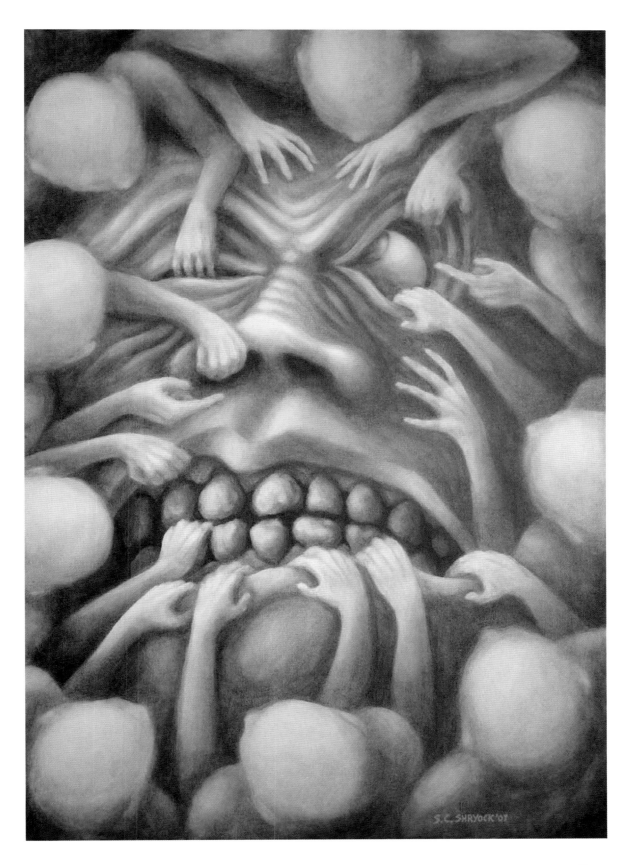

Awake
©2007

Noah Grossman
Age 26
Brooklyn, New York

A quiet hum. A soft white noise.
A loud white noise. An off-white noise.
A buzz abuzz. An idle vacuum one story up.
My brain microwaved. The unignorable endless note
of the world's longest bow
dragged across a one-stringed violin.
The static of Lenny Bruce's microphone.

My body's frequency grudgingly adjusts
to accommodate a generator bumping smoothly
below the floor. A blender mincing my constitution.
A tiny kettle screeching beneath my bed.
A far-off tire perpetually skidding
across my gray matter's blacktop.
The breathy sigh of a Gorgon.
The scream from a fatally wounded police cruiser
crawling out of my ear drum, echoing
insomnia's persuasive whisper.
A turbine hushed in a bed spring factory.

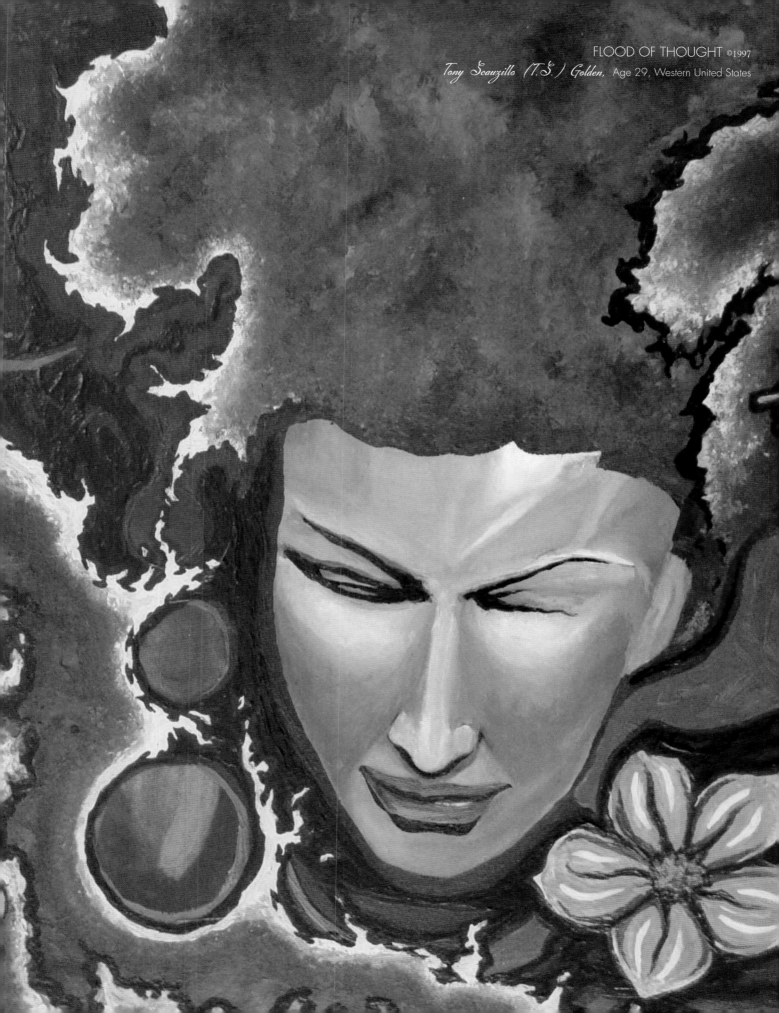

FLOOD OF THOUGHT ©1997
Tony Scauzillo (T.S.) Golden, Age 29, Western United States

SWEET VICTORY ©2007

Julia M. Shea, Age 38, Milwaukee, Wisconsin

it was a bad one. Painful in a way it had never been before but would continue to be for several years after.

He opened the door and peeked in, "Are you alright?"

I open my eyes briefly and lift my head from the bathroom floor to squint in his direction, "I'm going to die."

He sighed, "You're not going to die."

"How do you know? You aren't the one whose head is about to explode."

"Did you take your medicine?"

"Too late now. Doesn't work once the migraine is full blown. I just need to be left alone here to die. Please turn off the light, it's burning my pupils."

Wisely, he said nothing, turned off the light and shut the door. He was angry, but arguing with me was no fun if all I did was lie on the bathroom floor and ignore him. He blamed me for making him leave a friend's party early. Technically, it was my fault. I hadn't been feeling well all day and I refused to drink at the party because I knew it would make things worse. My not drinking agitated him. Everyone else was drinking and he was embarrassed that his girlfriend wouldn't because of a "headache." I would wish one of these on him so he could understand and sympathize with my pain, except this wasn't something you wish on anyone.

I had spent the night sitting in an overstuffed armchair, slouched down slightly so I could rest my head on the back without drawing too much attention to myself. I tried to smile and laugh with his friends while my head throbbed harder and harder. They kept offering me aspirin and joking that vodka on the rocks was just what I needed. All of them were clueless. By 10 p.m., the pain was so severe I could barely stand up straight. The room was spinning and my vision blurred and shifted with my pulse. When the nausea washed over me, I was on my way to the car, with or without him.

He took me home, not because he was truly concerned, but because he wasn't going to look like a jerk. I heard all about how crazy this was and how much I embarrassed him. "It's only a headache." I wish I could have thrown up in his lap.

Generally, I can only ride in a car comfortably with a migraine if I'm driving. By then that night, I was far too nauseous to drive, so I had to find a way to make it home without tossing my dinner into the front seat. This would have been easier if he hadn't been angry. He was driving fast, stopping hard, and turning wildly. Did I mention that migraines give me motion sickness? I slid to the floor of the car and put my head on the seat.

I couldn't decide whether I wanted him to keep driving fast to get me home or slow down so I didn't vomit. I was forever asking him to slow down and then to speed back up. The car seat was spinning. I closed my eyes, feeling my legs begin to cramp. It seemed like years before we pulled into the driveway.

He almost had to carry me into the kitchen because I was too dizzy to get there myself. I crawled up the stairs to the bathroom where I planned to spend eternity.

I bet I have lost several months of my life flat on my back because of a migraine. I went home sick from work, I didn't eat, and I cancelled plans. All I could do was sleep, but yet I couldn't. Every move, no matter how slight, sent new waves of pain pounding through my head. Sometimes it hurt to blink.

When it became clear to me that this wasn't just a phase I was going through, I decided I was not letting go of my life because of a headache. No matter how much I hated people calling it "just a headache," I knew I had to look at it that way to realize I didn't have to take it. The time I spent looking at migraines as a disease, I had felt powerless to heal myself and every couple of weeks, I spent several consecutive days in bed. By looking at migraines as just a headache, I was able to convince myself I could get rid of the pain. I began fighting back.

I started reading books like *Living Well With Migraine Disease and Headaches*, by Teri Robert and *What Your Doctor May Not Tell You About Migraines*, by Alexander Mauskop and Barry Fox. I tried feverfew, cold compresses, Excedrin for Migraine, magnesium and B vitamin supplements (believed to be lacking in migraine sufferers), and every prescription migraine medicine known to man. I bought into every marketed gismo that came out from compresses that actually stuck to your head to a lip balm-type tube claiming you could "rub away" your pain. I went through allergy testing/medications and a CT scan to be sure I didn't have sinus problems or another cause of my head pain.

As I stumbled along, I would often cry myself to sleep, begging God to make it stop. Many times, I asked him to come get me if I was going to have to deal with this pain for the rest of my life. I would rather have died than looked into the future with migraines.

Now, years later, I've got my migraines under control most of the time. I changed doctors and have finally gotten some ideas that are providing relief. She changed my birth control pills to a brand that continues to provide estrogen all the way through the cycle. I'm now taking a blood pressure medication known for success in preventing migraine attacks. Avoiding dairy and chocolate seem to help as well and I try my best to do that (but I love cheese and chocolate!). Stress is a big trigger for me and I try my best to keep out of stressful situations and calm myself down as quickly as possible.

It's been a long battle and I still get nasty headaches once in a while, but for the most part, I'm able to keep going through my day and ignore the pain. They aren't gone completely, but migraines don't take whole days away from me anymore.

I celebrate that as a victory every day. ☙

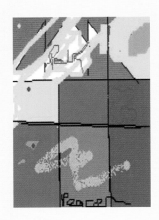

Pieces of Life ©2007

How do you put on paper the words to describe this pain,
This intense throbbing with no relief?
What do we do to block this path to agony —
Take this pill or that, What will help, What's the cause of this?
Why in blinding pain do we have to battle with a blister pack to yield the pill?
And how dare insurance companies limit relief
To just a few pills a month – profit is their only care.
Please, can't someone find the reason
That we must miss pieces of our lives?
And say more than "avoid wine and cheese."
Why don't experts have a handle on this, the answer, the key?
A day without a headache – Wow, maybe a few days without pain,
Then Pow, here we go again.
Those hours of life we lose can never be reclaimed.
My heart goes out to all who share these questions
As we survive the horrid days and cherish the good.

In the quilts I make, the colors of love and pain emerge,
Vibrating yellows and bright reds scream pain, blues and soft greens for gentle peace.
Connecting and blending, the fragments of our lives are like the parts of the quilt,
Living with all the colors, pain and peace, oh, how we treasure those beautiful pieces.

Linda Ann Crane
Age 61
Swartz Creek, Michigan

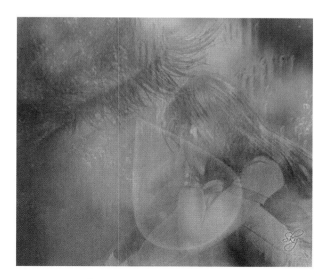

Sky ©2007 Age 42, West Virginia

Just for a Day ©2007

In this darkness,
I wonder when I will be set free
to laugh and smile,
hug and kiss,
dance and dream.

Sometimes I feel as if it will never come.

I know in time this darkness will set me free,
so I can
laugh and smile,
hug and kiss,
dance and dream, even if it's just for a day.

Linda Rae Stockton
Age 47
Portland, Oregon

"I never give up hope that the light of freedom is within my reach."

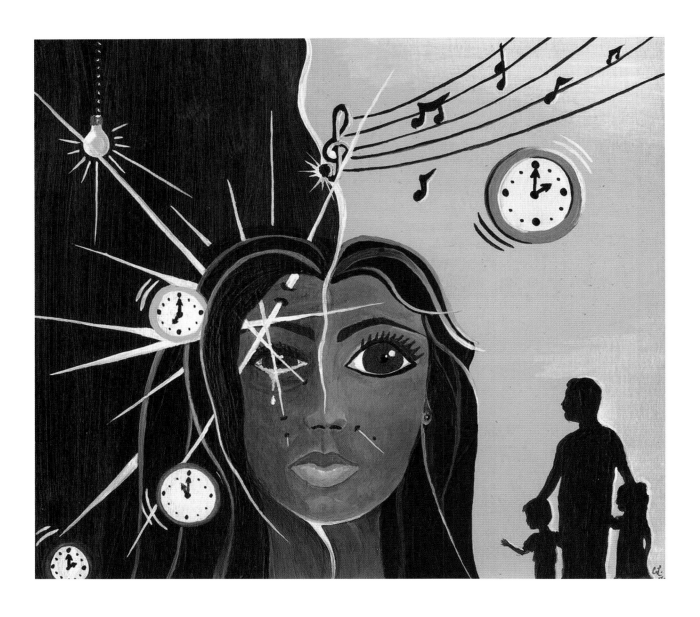

Mommy's Got a Headache ©2007

I have suffered from migraines for about 20 years, ever since I hit puberty. For me, the hardest part of living with migraines is trying to care for my daughter when I'm not feeling well. As a stay-at-home mom, I can't call in sick — I have to provide 24/7 coverage. I always muster through our day, often watching TV all day curled up on the couch together. Thank God for cable, especially the Disney channel and Noggin. Mickey Mouse can provide company for my daughter while I provide a simple physical presence. We get through the day with me glancing at the clock constantly, counting down the minutes until my husband gets home from work and I can go to bed alone. The only time I call for help is if I am so incapacitated that I can't stand to get up or I start vomiting from the pain. At that point, I throw in the towel and call for backup.

There is no worse feeling than believing you are a horrible mother who cannot care for your child — to not know from one day to the next whether or not you will be able to provide for your child in the manner she deserves. It makes me feel like a failure.

When I feel at my worse, I go lie down in my dark bedroom. My daughter comes in to say goodnight. She lays her chubby, sticky hand on my forehead and tells my husband, "Ssh! Mommy's got a headache!" She pulls the blanket up to my chin and gives me a sloppy kiss. Such love! Hope kindles in my heart that maybe I'm not such a terrible mother and tomorrow will be a better day.

Anchor ©2007

I want to fly high up in the sky leaving the ground far below me
Soaring and free
Away from this body wracked with pain
Beating from a tempo that no one else can hear
It won't let me leave, it won't let me fly
It has left me caged, anchored in this tomb of darkness,
solitude and quiet
      Will it never end
      So I can be a creature of light and life again

Essay & poem written by
Melissa Boots
Age 34, Lititz, Pennsylvania

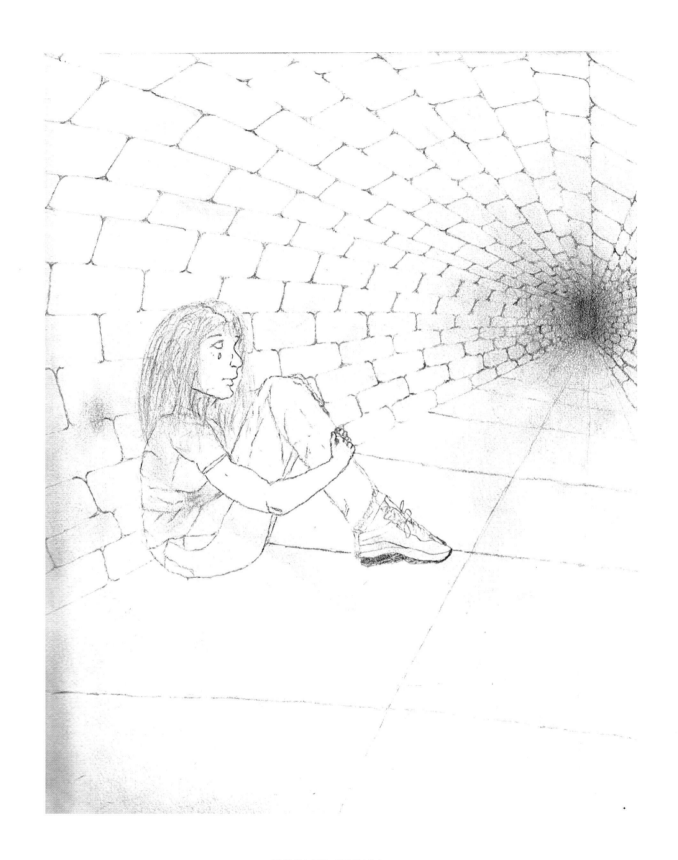

PRISONER OF PAIN ©2001

Jennifer A. Noland, Age 24, Fairbanks, Alaska

"I was about 18 when I made this sketch of a girl sitting in an endless tunnel from which there is no escape. It shows the hopelessness I was feeling about ever finding a way to function in everyday life with the migraines I was experiencing. I felt trapped by pain so intense that all I could do was lie down in a dark room until it went away."

Prisoner to an Inescapable Pain ©2007

The sudden aura:
It is my own, you could not detect it.
Waves of nausea sweep over me and send out a sure warning.
"Drink or eat NOW or you'll be sorry," it threatens.

"Take your pills, close your eyes. Take your pills, clear your head."
I am stuck, sitting on a bus, departing from school, age 17...
And I am in this, for better or worse – and forever.
How did such simple tasks turn to such trying feats?

Surrounded by smiling passengers, all unaware of my invisible hell.
I search for the prescription pills to halt a certain storm.
I swallow them, with no water — time is of the essence.
The large red capsules twist awkwardly down my throat, never in perfect form.

Meanwhile, sounds set fire to a pounding in my head.
It can only be extinguished by later vomiting, then sleeping soundly.
Soon my own coughing hurts to be heard.
And yes of course, *I've tried to escape you, but you've found me.*

I am your prisoner and your guinea pig — why so often and why now?
Too much pain for the questions, too much pain for the answers...
The bus stops and I raise my head and rush to the door.
And then my world is an excruciating blur, too complicated for any words.

I hurry, sobbing, to my house — and yes that hurts; even that hurts.
Temples throbbing, eyes barely open, I'm unaware when I throw my stuff to the floor.
I go straight to the toilet; yellow bile rushes to leave my system.
It may seem disgusting, but *I am so aware of you that all else is ignored.*

Flash forward:
Age 24, For you, I have to leave my job early sometimes.
And despite all else, I know what I may have to do.
Pull over and stop everything. Pull over and close my eyes.
So I can momentarily conquer you.

I will never have all the answers, but I rely on simple "helpers..."
Food, water, pills and sleep allow me to be myself once again.
So with my army of little efforts I will remain ready and waiting.
...Until then, my *forever-"friend,"* Until then.

J. Johnson
Age 24, Los Angeles, California

Demon in My Head ©2007

Darkness has descended.
I close my eyes because I must.
Thunder booms with each breath.
Inside my head there lives a demon
who torments me when I am doing my best
to ignore him.
With each tentative smile and every pain-free day
I feel him lurking in wait
for my back to turn
and my guard to be down.
And then he attacks.
And I am rendered motionless
soundless, light-less and joyless.
I lie in purposeful shadows
because brightness screams
and noise destroys
and the only thing that brings respite
is a blanketed hiding-out
where even sleep is no escape.
The worst of this brutal punishment is,
No one understands.
They wonder if I am exaggerating.
They narrow their eyes in hidden suspicion
when I use this excuse for the millionth time.
No one knows the extent of my suffering
so I suffer alone until the demon retreats
until the darkness lifts
until the deadly storm passes by
and I can do more than lie in frustrated wait
wishing death upon the demon in my head.

Jessica Vitelli, Age 32, Newton, Massachusetts

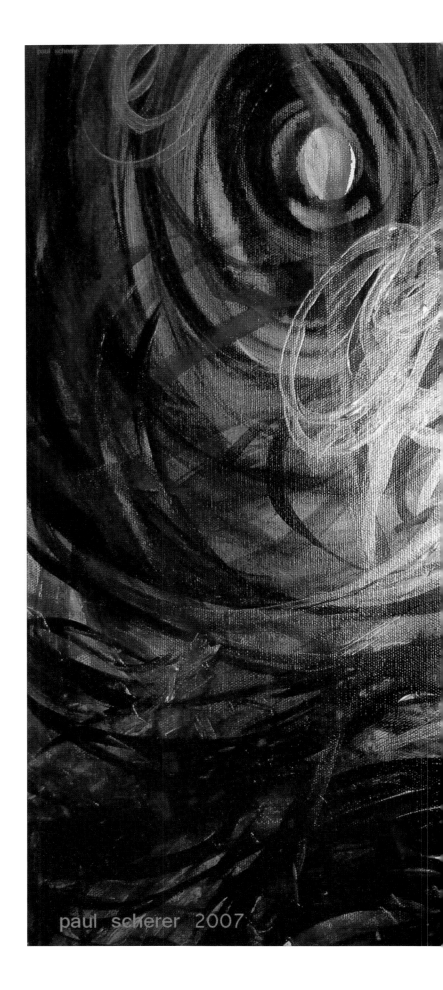

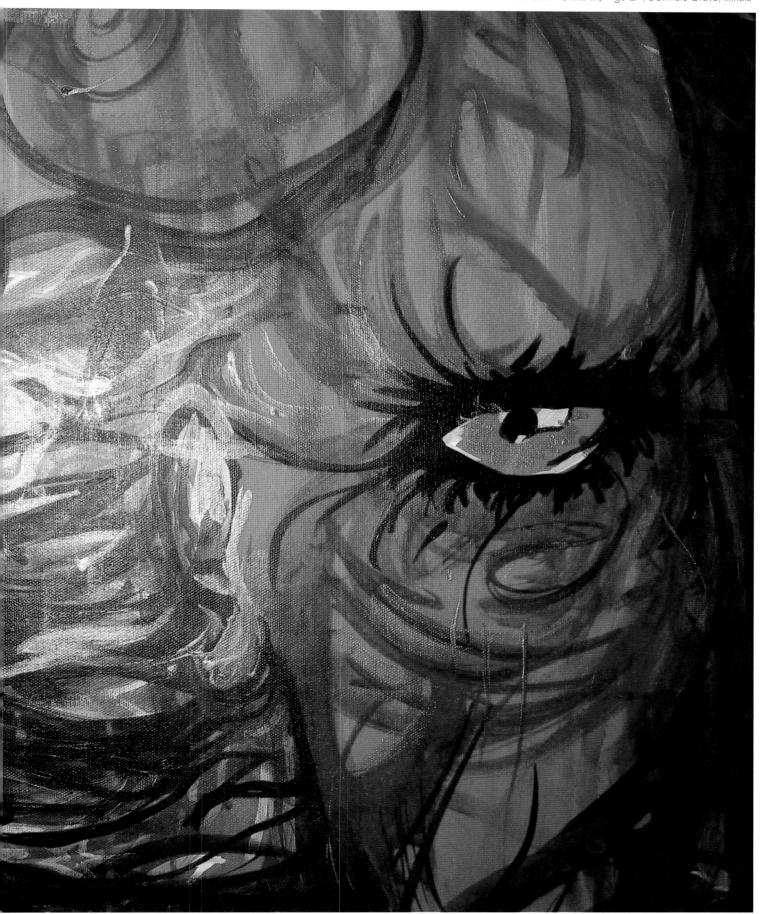

the quiet magician ©2007

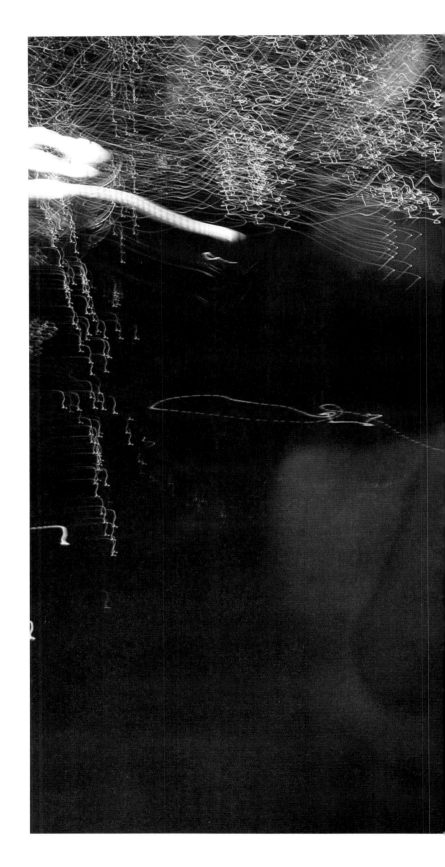

you outshone the stage lights the arguments
the bitter stances
for or against the calculations the half rememberings
the to-do list the do I want this

quiet.

how slyly you press with your abstract symphony
your choreographing of the color wheel
to boast more and more and without any order
of which I can stand to see or to guess at

but when your warring notes fade
when the sun you have been in league with
steps politely a little away I see what you had to say
and simply it is that

I had forgotten where I live.

bone muscle blood to walk to run get out of my head
to pull back the blinds
to honor with every sense all that is delectable
and vibrant without and within.

Valerie Joy Kalynchuk
Age 32, Toronto, Ontario, Canada

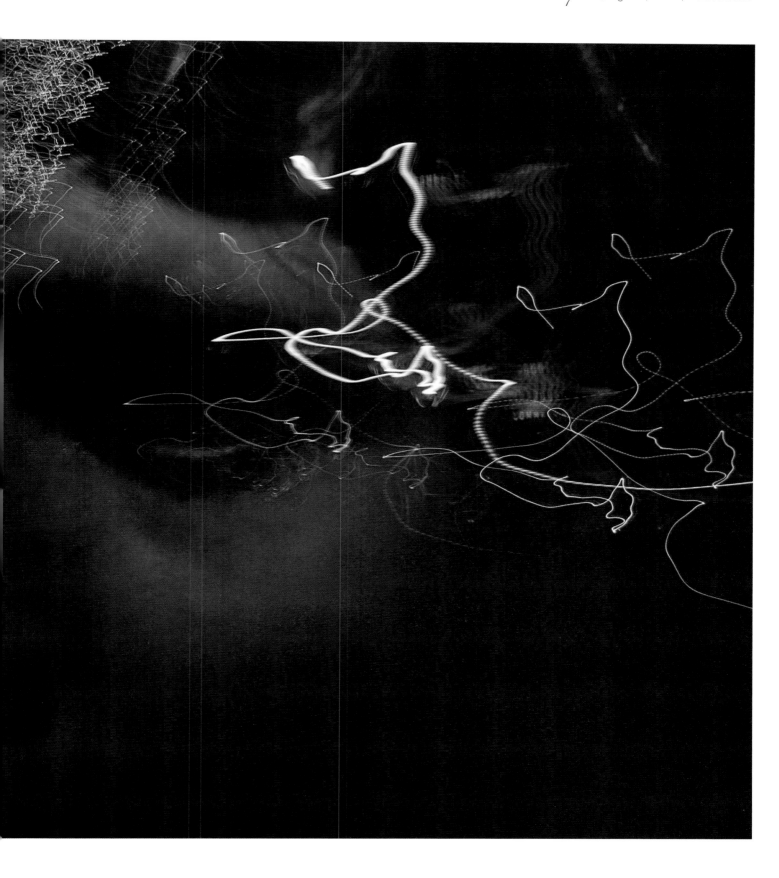

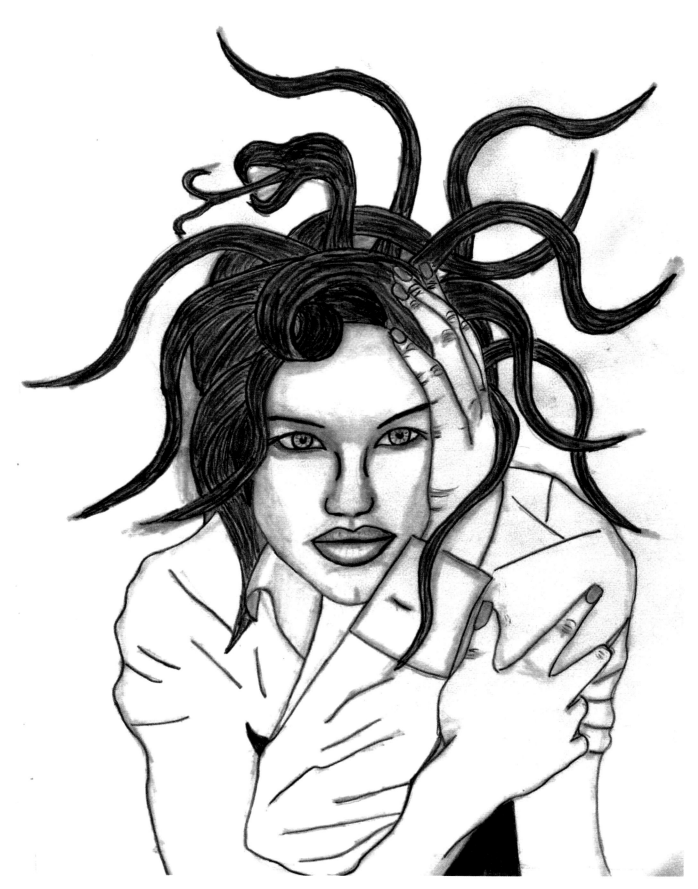

Migraineur ©2007

Lolita Paiewonsky, Cambridge, Massachusetts

and so ....

this python in my head
it kicks like a monster child
it moves around to other places at times
like it is chasing something
chasing after something
  maybe it is trying to find a way out,
out of my head
out of my body

ii

standing is murder
walking - ever so slowwwwly - is torrrrrture
riding in a boyfriend's car - cataclyyyyssssmic
finally reaching safe haven - a bed
easing into a prone position
the hammer's striking does not abate
until, finally, who-knows-how-long-it-took
the horsepilldrug kicks in and sleep tiptoes in as if not to disturb the dragon's tail

iii

don't.
do not awaken
remain prone
stay asleep
asleep in safehaven, arms of morpheo

 iv.

do not dream, either
it is dangerous to dream
the python is monitoring the r.e.m.s

v.

the horse and the python wrestle
not a pretty sight
the wrestling 'tween snake and steed
Faust duped?
Eurydice enticed?
what would Migraineur give   trade   barter   do
to break free
be free

vi.

one impossible volcanic eruption
The Final Shot of Pain
fast yet unendurable
Or,
a Gentle Easing Away Pain
vaseline extrication
from the grip of the relentless muscle mass
endurable to the ecstasy at the end of the tunnel
(but how long? and what if —·'
     what if, oh, unsayable thing,
     it was all a trick, and the torture interminable —')

vii.

drifting through sheets of pelting rain, rain
hailing down in *adagios*
     consciousness
                    reality
                    dreaming
                    fretting
is it day or night ?
     where is the moon that inhabits both morning and twilight

viii.

the rain, steady now,
filters through a window
tears through slits of my eyes, eyes
I am afraid to open
     black or grey or red beneath frowns that
          tighten or
          let go like blinking eyelids through which
scores of ravens escape

ix.

sleep walking
awake walking through years
into bushes, highways of real
     grownup headaches with worries for pythons
until the real pythons return again

"As far as I can recall, I was first stricken with migraines — and diagnosed as such — during my third year of college while spending the summer in Chicago. The intensity and frequency subsided some years later. Twenty years after the onset, I continue to suffer headaches. Nothing, however, as any migraineur is painfully aware, approaches the brunt of A Migraine Headache. When I received notice of this anthology and wondered if I might submit, I was unprepared for the deluge of emotion… the vivid, frightful memories… the release and peace when the python rested."

©2007 *Melissa S. Treacy*
Age 26, Eagleville, Pennsylvania

Children don't always understand things. We teach them everything they know, feel and comprehend in life. Unfortunately, teaching them pain is a part of that learning experience. We have to help them to understand what pain is, what it means and how it affects us all.

Pain is a difficult lesson to teach. Children know that they have felt pain. They understand the word. Pain is getting a shot at the doctor's office. Pain is scraping a knee at the playground. Pain is when Fluffy the rabbit died last summer. Those things all mean pain.

But since pain is something you cannot touch or see, it is a hard emotion to explain. Pain can vary from the physical wound, to a deep-down heartache. Pain can be immense, or sometimes soon forgotten. It can scar you for life, always under the surface. Or, it can be a momentary lapse in the daily routine.

Migraines are just one form of pain. When that pain strikes, its sufferer knows it. It is unstoppable, unannounced and crippling. It controls the life of all involved. Time must stop until the pain subsides. The pain takes over.

This is a hard concept for even an adult to understand, but a child may take even longer. How do you explain that mommy needs the lights to stay off? Mommy needs it to be very quite. Please, turn off that television; it is too loud today. A toddler simply stares in disbelief. How could such a thing take mommy over?

But, thankfully, children are also resilient. They love unconditionally. While they do not understand, they will do everything they can to comply. Even at the tender age of two, he can feel compassion. He can know that it is hurting mommy.

He can understand pain.

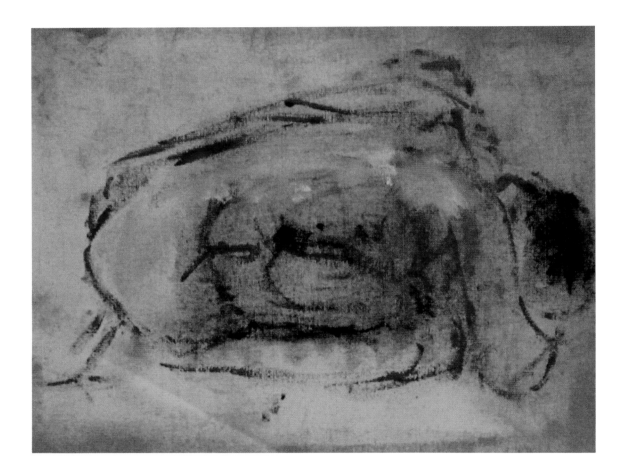

Marginal

©2007

Fran Merlie
Age 22
Pennsylvania

My mother woke triumphant,
the champ of another bout

against the fingers wrapped
around her brain, entrenched

and pinching, squeezing coarse blood
in stabbing pumps around her head.

Relieved, she stood, her eyes
now dry of tears, her face relaxed,

her nostrils growing wide
for oxygen free of the weight

it had carried. The shades will rise
and she will spend the morning

reading Joan Didion,
who suffers a similar pain

but whose writing is free
from unwelcome words

that would weigh down the prose
like the blood that filled my mother's head.

The morning will deepen into afternoon,
where headaches are distant, painless

memories hidden in the gaps
between words, between pages.

A STUDENT OF MIGRAINES ©2007

Sharon Davis, Age 55, Trabuco Canyon, California

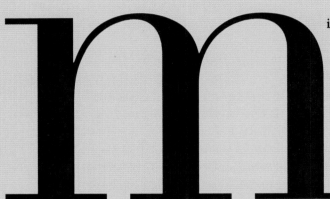

igraines have shadowed and shaped my life for 10 years. I didn't want to give them that power. They just took it. I have come closer to the brink of despair than I would have thought possible for someone of my basically upbeat temperament. I got a good look at its bleak, gray landscape and I don't ever want to go back. I'm in a better place now. I'd like to say I did something right, but frankly I think I just got lucky. Time is on my side in this war — getting older has its perks. I learned a lot along the way about coping with pain, about what is important to me, and, believe it or not, about gratitude.

My mother had classic migraines as a young woman, complete with aura, or visual disturbances, that forced her to lie down in a dark room until they went away. Her mother before her suffered from what she so very accurately called her "sick headaches." I was blithely unconcerned by these stories, convinced I had escaped that fate. After all, I reached my 40s with nothing more than the occasional, albeit intense, tension headache that I treated with my pain reliever of choice, Excedrin. Ah, the lovely rush of caffeine! However, beginning in my early to mid-40s, a number of factors began to accumulate, creating, unbeknownst to me, the perfect storm.

The most significant of these factors was perimenopause. I didn't even know that such a thing existed until I was halfway through it. When I was around 44, however, I began to get these strange headaches that wouldn't go away. When I think back on my naive, puzzled response to those early migraines, my complete lack of comprehension, my utter certainty that it was just a little road bump that would smooth out very shortly, I want to go back and give myself a hug. Because now I know what lay ahead, and just how many bumps, potholes, mud bogs and dirt roads I would have to navigate.

Basically, they were menstrual migraines. The least understood and least manageable migraine there is. They came roughly once a month, unrelentingly, and they lasted from 48 to 72 hours no matter what I did to try to control them. The pain was on the right side of my head, slightly up and behind the right eye. It affected the right side of my neck and my right shoulder as well. Anyone who has had one knows how hard it is to describe to someone who has only experienced a tension headache: the general malaise, the nausea, the fatigue. They made me feel sick all over. I usually tried to power through day one, sticking as much to my normal routine as possible. On day two I would take to my bed unless it was absolutely necessary that I be upright. On day three, as the pain began to recede, fatigue and a kind of blank feeling would set in. Then it would be over for a while: usually three-and-a-half to four weeks; sometimes, miraculously, six weeks; sometimes, crushingly, two weeks.

Those were my migraines. They made me sick, they made me cry, they left me exhausted. They made my family sad and frustrated. The migraine sufferer does not suffer alone. My husband and I started our family a little later than most people. I was 38 and he was 35 when we married (first marriage for both of us). I was 39 and 42 when my two children were born. I had wonderful pregnancies, easy births, beautiful children. I am a profoundly lucky

woman, let me say that right now. It is the love for and from that admirable husband and those beautiful children that has seen me through this.

When the headaches began, my daughter was five and my son was two. So picture me in my 40s, beginning to slow down a bit, with two very young, active children. Now imagine the arrival of my in-laws who took up residence in our back bedroom for what was supposed to be a brief transition to their new lives as retirees but was in fact a permanent arrangement, with time off for long visits to their other children, until the end of their lives. Add to this mix the fact that at the beginning of this period, my husband was experiencing some uncertainty and instability in his work life, and money was tight. What have I just described? A terrifying recipe for the onset of migraines? No. In fact, I have just described the lives of millions of women. The fact of the matter is, we all have stress in our lives. I do not name all these factors for sympathy. I got plenty of that. The people in my life were always assuming the headaches had something to do with them. That is precisely the point. The headaches did not have anything to do with them. It is really tempting, when people keep suggesting that they are the reason for your pain, or the tight money or the tight living quarters are the reason for your pain, you poor thing, it is quite tempting to slide into that point of view. To blame. Nevertheless, I always knew in my heart that stress was not causing these headaches. Is it harder to cope with stress when you have a migraine? Absolutely. It put additional stress on me to feel that I was letting the people I loved down, to appear to be the kind of person who takes to her bed with a headache when things get a little tough. I knew that was not who I was.

So none of those factors caused the headaches. They did, however, make it more difficult for me and everyone else to deal with the two or three days a month I was useless. I remember one time my mother-in-law made the comment, "Maybe your headaches will go away when we move out." Being on day two of one of my migraines made me tactless and, without thinking, I quickly replied, "I wish it was that easy." The look on her face told me I had said the wrong thing.

What is so hard to explain to non-migraineurs is that the headaches have a life of their own. They have their own frightening logic, and they dictate your life accordingly. I have thought about colorful comparisons. Migraines are the bullies who continue to twist your arm long after, tears streaming down your face, you have cried "uncle," the wicked stepmother who always finds another job for you and never lets you rest, a blood-red fog you struggle to see through, terrified of losing your way. None of these works, none of them fit. Because in the end, what is so scary about a migraine is precisely that it is not an external force. External forces can be controlled or avoided. Migraines come from within. They are the incomprehensible betrayal of an otherwise healthy body.

So, what to do, how to cope? There is no miracle cure. Once I accepted that (and that took a while), I was able to slowly build my own little personal arsenal to fight the beast. Medication can play a big role for some people. For me, personally, I found that simple treatments were more effective and sustainable. Ibuprofen would give me as much actual pain relief as any other prescription or OTC medication. Now, mind you, it is not a lot of pain relief, but anything is better than nothing.

To quickly summarize my hard-won pain management routine, gleaned over years of trial and error: what works for me now is ibuprofen, bed rest, patience, good books, a sense of humor, love, gratitude and hope. In roughly that order. However, in order to actually have some of those things to draw on in the midst of the pain (most notably hope) there is some work that has to be done in between the migraines. For me, this included keeping a journal. It was really just a calendar where I kept track of the migraines and made notes about diet and activity that might have some bearing. I was also an avid reader, reading every book, magazine and newspaper article I could find about the subject. I was very open to alternative therapies and used meditation and relaxation to control pain. All these things gave me a sense of control over what was happening to me. I can't stress how important that was for me, because giving me some control gave me hope, and hope is the antidote to despair.

About gratitude — you read a lot about gratitude in self-help books these days. There is a reason for that. It works. When you focus on that for which you are grateful, it multiplies. But where does gratitude fit into the hellish world of migraines? How is it possible to be grateful in the midst of the grim reality of a migraine? Here I must quote Joan Didion, who, by her own account, has suffered from migraines four or five times a month since she was eight years old. In her beautiful and elegant essay, "In Bed," from *The White Album*, she says: "For when the pain recedes, ten or twelve hours later, everything goes with it, all the hidden resentments, all the vain anxieties… There is a pleasant convalescent euphoria. I open the windows and feel the air, eat gratefully, sleep well. I notice the particular nature of a flower in a glass on the stair landing. I count my blessings."

Allow me to count a few blessings. I'm sure there were many days when my husband, Mike, came home from a hard day at work thinking the last thing he wanted to face was a wife with a migraine. He seldom if ever betrayed that attitude. He would sit down and listen to me complain, for the hundredth time, about the pain. He would offer sympathy and encouragement, and I would feel a little better because of it. He was always on the lookout for newspaper articles and other kinds of information about migraines for me; he encouraged me to try alternative therapies, like acupuncture, and never flinched at the cost or wackiness; and, bless him, he knew when to leave me the heck alone. He knew instinctively that all of these things were like strands of hope that I could string together into a rope to make a bridge across the chasm. I am very grateful to him.

I used to get very sad thinking about my children growing up with a mother who had monthly migraines. What would they remember, I wondered: a sad, tired woman lying on the couch? Were they frightened? Were they resentful? Of course, I can't really answer all those questions, but I can tell you this. They were really, really sweet. My son, Kenny, loved to give me foot rubs, and let me tell you, they were the best. My daughter, Sarah, would lie with me and chat and read, and make cards for me. I have very peaceful memories of those times, because I always made a promise to myself when I felt a migraine coming on that I would be very patient with my children and not take it out on them. So, ironically, I was frequently kinder to them then than I was when I was "normal." Just as important to me as those memories, however, are the times when I was forced to close the door to all visitors, and they were free to not fuss over me. They were still resilient enough, still confident enough in the overall health and safety of their family, to slip into the innocent oblivion of children, to rush outside to play with friends and be, I sincerely hope, truly carefree.

If my friend, Liz, never got sick of me showing up for our lunch date with that strained "I've got a migraine" look on my face, she never showed it. I made it a point to keep those dates, because I always left feeling better. She was a great tonic for me. Friends are important in the support structure for migraineurs, but there is a simple rule: spend time with positive, upbeat people; stay away from negative, downbeat people.

Finally, I am grateful to my mother-in-law. Yes, there were times when I wished she would just go away, as cruel as that sounds. I am a person who craves a fair amount of solitude, especially when I have a migraine. When my in-laws were with us, they were always at home, there was no escape unless I left the house.

However, having said that, let me say that they were very good people who raised an excellent son. I also now realize what an important part of my support system they were. I am grateful to my mother-in-law for the times she picked up the slack with my kids and in the kitchen. I miss her very much.

So why am I able to speak in the past tense about my migraine experience? First of all, let me make a confession: I still have migraines. Now, however, I get them every three to six months instead of every three to six weeks. I believe there are two reasons for this. I finally went through menopause and have not had a period for almost two years. Also, and I believe this is a big also, at about the same time that my periods stopped, I began to take blood pressure medication. So which is it? I honestly don't know. It might be a combination of both. I know that I have gotten a migraine when I have forgotten to take my blood pressure medication for several days running. However, because I do believe that hormones played a large role in my migraine experience, I also strongly believe that no periods equals no (or fewer) migraines.

Frankly, I can live with a little medical mystery when I'm on this side of it. Now when I get a migraine, I lie down and have a rest. While I am resting, I meditate on how profoundly grateful I am for all the days, weeks and months I can now string together with no migraines. I am also truly grateful for all I have learned. ৩৩

The Angel of Migraines ©2007

Eugenia Toledo-Keyser
Age 61, Seattle, Washington

I

Death has come here
Disguised as a migraine again
Hidden in the folds of life
In the night, in silence,
In the pages I write
Like ray and thunder
From a hell of slow dying.

The dark angel took me over,
A moment known only to itself to say:
"Here I am.
I have been following you for years
Like the shadow that can't be left at home.
Like oblivion, yes like oblivion
You no longer want to remember.
It's useless to turn your head away:
I'm so close you can't see me coming,
I'm outside you and within.
You want to believe
That you will be healthy without me;
But, no, not a single day
Nor the hours when you want to stop me,
To fight me, to trick me or forget me.
Here I am, can't you feel me?
Close your eyes, close the curtains,
Close carefully the door,
Remain in the darkness and the silence.
Here I am."

And now, I ask myself,
What mysterious force does this?
What kind of destiny?
Why is here suddenly, uninvited, this horrible guest?
What made that sheet of paper fall from the table?

And now, pressing my temples,
Something like blood pulses, throbbing pain,
That circulates inside my head,
And I know that the crooked letters
I now write,
Shakier, weak, more faint,
No longer come from my hand alone.

II

And you, only you, know that death
Is the choked words, the groans
And the throbbing pain I suffer
When I wrestle the Angel of Migraine.

Migraine is all this and more
That encircles me
Pulls me away from life,
And finally leaves me dizzy and
Hanging with an aura
That doesn't bleed.

III

If I keep you imprisoned,
And control you and hide you;
If I medicate you in the depths
Of my most intimate suffering,
If my death gives you another life
What will become of you?
Lugubrious Migraine,
When I must leave this body,
Untying this tangled knot,
You too will end and rest?

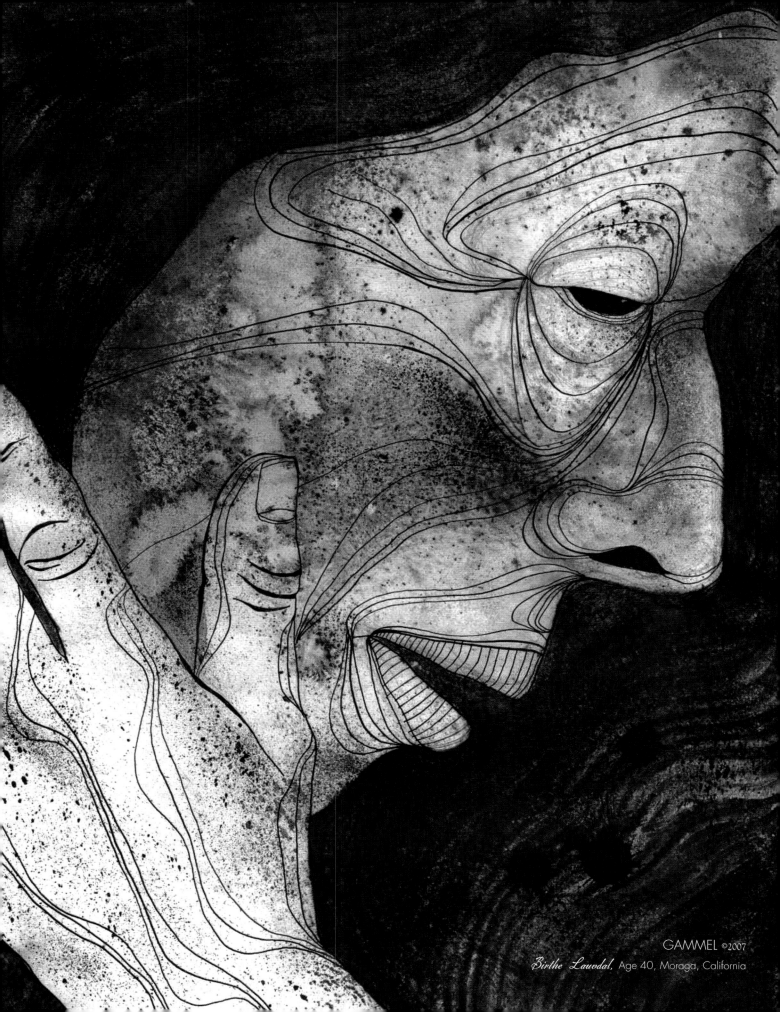

GAMMEL ©2007

Birthe Lauvdal, Age 40, Moraga, California

A Common Attack *or* Before Triptans
©1985

Jill Richards
Age 67
Great Malvern, England

Barbed arrows crucify the cranium
Punishing with piercing pain.
Daggers thrust at painful sockets
Forcing eyes to close.
Lances sear the neck.

I'm paying the price for yesterday's pleasure.
Retreat behind drawn curtains,
Agony, curled in sheets.

Invidiously, pain's downward onslaught advances
Puncturing the stomach
With wave after wave of nauseous eruption.
It penetrates the gut,
Tortured, the body screams evacuation.

Pain's battle rages,
Consolidating its inner onslaught
Remorselessly, unyieldingly, persistently
On the grey-mattered torture chamber.
Hour after hour, day after day
Head's shields thump, bang,
Bruised in the hard clash with pain's armour.

Between skirmishes, sleep anaesthetizes
The anguish of body and mind.
Outside, two, three or four, unlived days pass by.
Then one incredibly beautiful dawn
Chinks of light and sound are readmitted.

Breakfast soothes a battered body
To emerge weak, but victorious.
Yet again another attack is repulsed
And even after all these years
The defences believe there can never be another.

"This poem from the past recollects the severity of migraine attacks when my then-young family crept around our house because Mum was so ill."

AS I OPENED MY EYES ©2007

Angela Carlo, Age 27, Oakland, California

"My mother has suffered migraines for years and the brain is a very strong theme in my art."

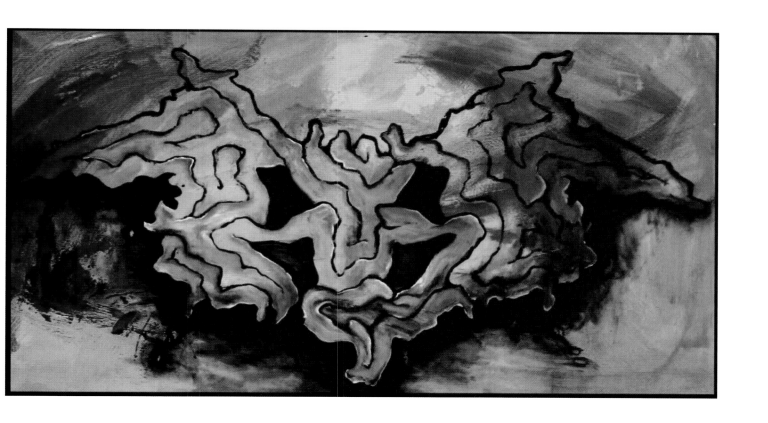

"My mother has suffered migraines for years and the brain is a very strong theme in my art."

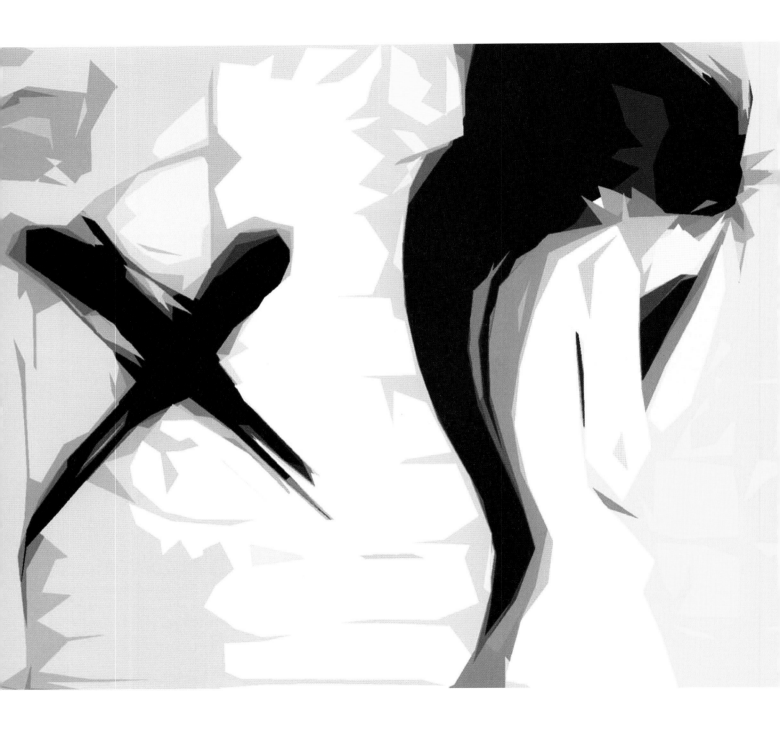

BEATEN BY WORDS ©2007

Tim Dankanich, Age 32, Philadelphia, Pennsylvania

"When all open space becomes filled with static pressure and vertigo distractions, when every little sound turns into ugly children kicking and screaming on the interior of one's skull, the echoes sometime sound like, 'Are you okay? Are you alright? What's wrong?' The minutes seem to drag and file their fingernail bodies across the chalkboard face of the clock. The only thing one can do is wait. Wait until the suffering is over. If you squint your eyes as though you were in the worst pain you can imagine, the image becomes clearer. 'Are you okay? Are you alright? What's wrong?'"

Lessons
©2007

Michael Clyne
Age 23
Bethpage, New York

There are warnings you might learn
to recognize and dread
and in retrospect you might discern
the shape that stuffed your head

The face that smirked atop the crazed
behemoth of your pain
the emblem that etched a space
your weightless words cannot retain

You might find wicked Christmas lights
between the dark room and your eyes
nailed as yellow to your sight
as ribbons round your oak trees' thighs

But despite its sharp consequence
the vision brings no understanding
no metaphor could merge with sense
the sign and its shrill meaning

It's not a question of complexity
a matter just of awful size
all your senses intersecting with
a point too enormous to describe

Your cache of fears and memories
will need to be postponed
for the lone lesson that serenity
is born from weakness before hope

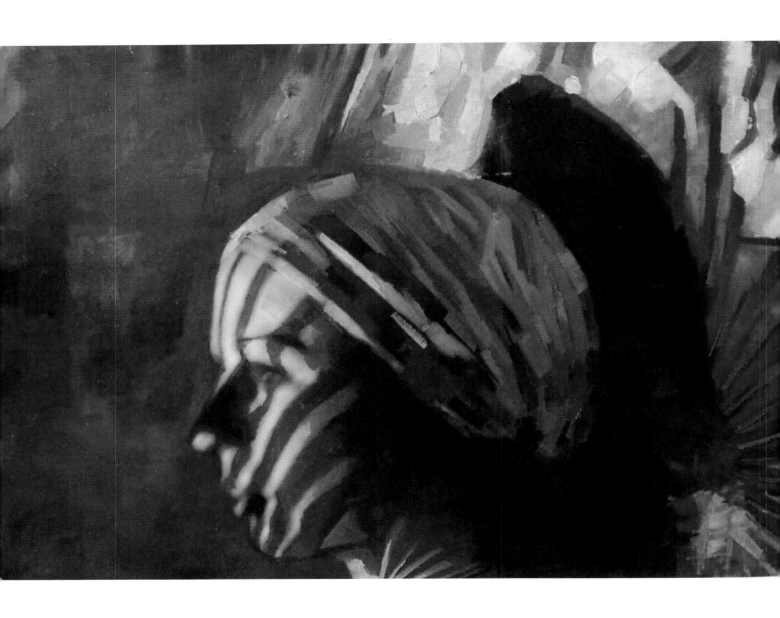

PAINTED PROJECTIONS ©2007

Debi Tonge, Age 35, San Francisco, California

"I think this image describes the intense pain that violently travels across my head and all one can do is be still and brave."

Thursday, 3 pm

©2007

Lauren Koblara
Age 26
West Brookfield, Massachusetts

I am huddled in my own cocoon
Hiding from a shard of light
That barely breaks the darkness
But is burning like the sun
I clench my eyes as tight as fists
And I tighten the vise

I am sheltered in my tiny cave
My breath echoes like thunder
My pulse is a loud drum beat
I hear the blood in my veins
Or at least I think that I can
And I swallow the cure

I am waiting for the melt-away
To feel each layer of pain
Slowly, surely fade to white
So I can regain myself
I inhale a determined breath
And return to the world

HEAD TRAUMA ©2007

Meagan Louise, Age 25, Oakland, California

"This photograph represents for me the pain of the migraines I have watched my best friend of 21 years live with for most of her life. Though I've never experienced the excruciating pain of a migraine, I imagine it to look somewhat like this."

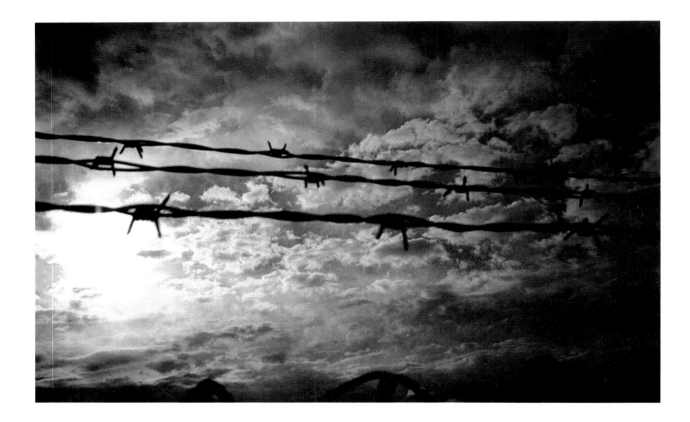

Rainmaker ©2007

It throbs and pulsates in the left side of my brain
Like an old Indian banging his drum waiting for rain
I wait for the silence that will keep me sane
I can't think at all never mind think straight
All I can do is ride it out, All I can do is wait
Feels like a war is going on inside my skull and I can't get to bed
I try and sleep but the pounding is too much for my head
I'd like to pick up a gun but I reach for the sleeping pills instead
I would never do it but at least it would be quiet if I were dead
I wish I could cut a hole and leak it out, sew it up with a needle and thread
But It would just come back stronger next time with weight like lead
I know there are others like me, I know you feel my pain
Just believe me when I say soon the Indian will bring the rain

Cory Piekarski
Age 27, Attleboro, Massachusetts

Stress sits in my shoulders
Crimping my posture
Tightening my stance
Always tense

My head pounds
Teeth clench
Scowling cannot be helped
The pain is constant

Turn off the lights
Tuck into bed
No noise, please
Nothing will help

It is a constant
Always painful
Never a warning
Always painful

Never a warning
For this horrible pain
Creeps up on you
Taking your day away

Pleading for sleep
Where there is no pain
Maybe tomorrow
It will be gone

© 2007 *Melissa S. Treacy*
Age 26, Eagleville, Pennsylvania

Migraine ©1994

A migraine is a touch of death, an inkling of the end.
When suffering in the midst of one you feel you'll never mend.
Death's fingers brush across one eye, grip becomes more fierce
And you retreat into a world of pain, as sharp nails pierce.
A day, two days, then slowly as undents this ball of woe
Normality returns. Inflated, life restored, you go.
Betwixt each visitation life is radiant, a boon,
Until death calls the next time round with paralysing tune.
So, when the end comes finally 't'will be a sweet release,
No waves of migraine ever more, just great, eternal peace!

Moira Vaughan
Age 61, Edinburgh, Scotland

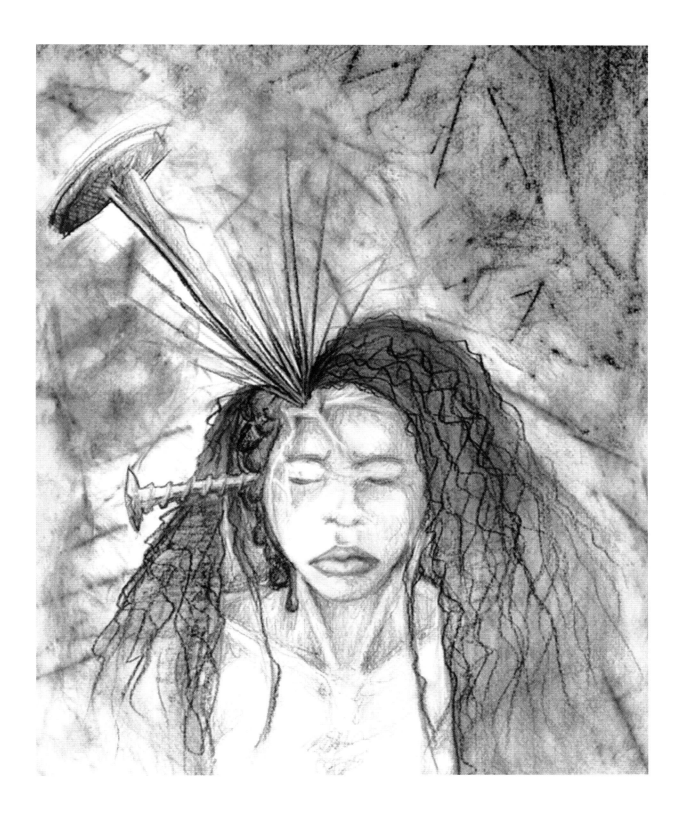

NEUROLOGICAL RECONSTRUCTION ©2007

Camille Waller, Age 20, Savannah, Georgia

"I have never been able to convey my experiences in writing and came to realize that my migraines have always been so severe and disorienting that no words could describe them. Consequently, I've conveyed a migraine visually in a charcoal and graphite drawing, with hopes that it will feed me the words it was made to speak."

My pain

Tightening

Lightning

Blinding

Binding

Lighting

Blighting

Gripping

Slipping

Swimming

Hotly

Swirling

Dervish

Of pain

Stabbing

Jabbing

Grabbing

Vicelike

Churning

Rumbling

Tumbling

Falling

Into the

Abyss

Migraine Drain
©2007

Christa Joyce
Age 49
London, England

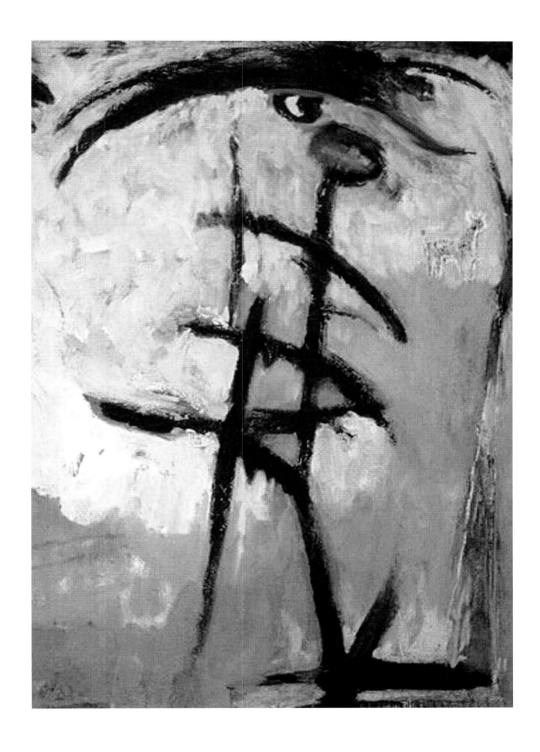

ME AND MY HEADACHE ©1995, Oil on Canvas 24" x 36"
Judi Pettite, Age 43, Oakland, California

"In the painting, I am the figure falling/flying helplessly over the stiff black armature in the foreground — centered, affronting, effectively pushing me out of the picture frame. The scene has a landscape background, the moon is rising in a twilight sky — reflective of the suspended state I experience trying to negotiate the unwieldy nature of a migraine."

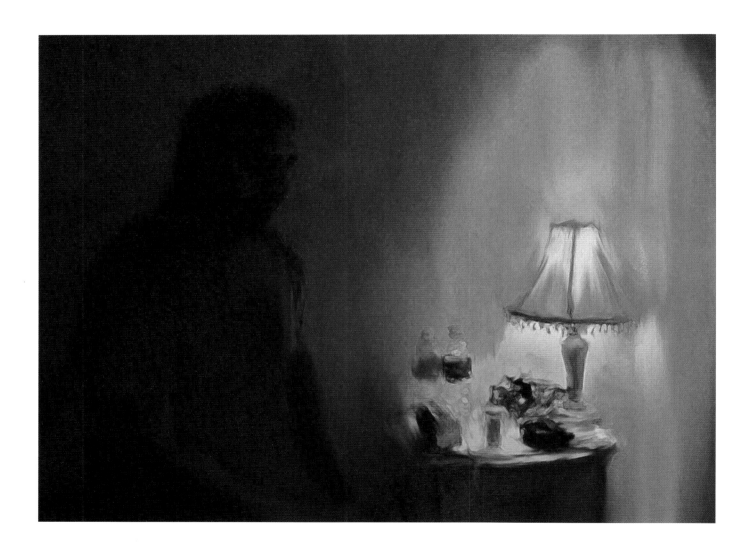

MIGRAINES, MARRIAGE, SUFFERING ©2007

Aimee Houser

> [M]y own adventure of suffering… can take on a meaning, the only meaning to which suffering is susceptible, in becoming a suffering for the suffering — be it inexorable — of someone else.
> — Emmanuel Levinas, "Useless Suffering," *The Provocation of Levinas: Rethinking the Other*, 1988

When it hits, I'm reminded of our joke: that we should paint the spare bedroom black. He stumbles to bed, and as he folds a towel over his eyes, we talk about how, again, we've forgotten to replace the mask we threw away after the cat's vomiting spree. I push the slats of the wood blinds, trying to stamp out light. He rolls to his side, pulls his legs up: an unreadable glyph, all right angles, stiff with pain. I offer things he doesn't want — a glass of water, a cold compress — but I don't know what else to do.

We both know what's coming: sleep for at least 12 hours as the symptoms of an active migraine wrack his body. Then, another day or so of sluggishness and bluesy feelings. He will take an NSAID when the first signs come over him: nausea, drowsiness, blinking and squinting to keep the light from stabbing his eyes like brilliant, hard-edged gems. But he will not take triptans; taking them may initiate cardiac events in people with risk factors. In his family, as in mine, heart problems are common, sometimes fatal.

While we were in graduate school in the late 1990s, my husband had a large gray Buick that he used to cart us and our circle of friends from pizza joint to bars to breakfast joint, and that we called "Nixon" after the beginning letters of its license plate, "NXN." But when alone in the car, we solemnly remembered the gift's source: his uncle, who died young of a heart attack. My father-in-law, brother of the uncle, also had heart disease in his late 40s, underwent successful bypass surgery. At that time, my husband was away at undergraduate school and thankfully knew little about it.

I see traces of that medical lineage when his eyelids begin drawing down. I know of no known connection between heart disease and migraines.

But through a trick more of my own family history than his, the two conditions are for me intimately bound up in one another. When I look into my husband's strained face, the wan pallor, I see the afterimage of my father, his face, in a Polaroid taken Christmas Day, 1982. He is standing with his brother, arm over shoulder, fraternal. Shadows encircle my father's heavy eyes; his cheeks are sallow and flat. A kind of transition is visible, I think now, between life and not-life, between the day's hope before and the day's hopelessness next, when paramedics will come, fruitlessly.

❧

On a recent migraine-free day, with not a single symptom in sight, I brought up the joke about the black room, suggesting we actually do it. Black walls and white furniture? A design statement, according to *Domino Magazine*. We could do something a little less Tim Burton and more farmhouse colonial, I suggested, a deep blue maybe.

"Paint a room black — blue?" my husband asked, fuzzily.

"You don't remember?"

"No," he replied.

"It's a joke we — or at least I thought we — have about painting a bedroom in a dark color so you have a light-free place to go when you get a migraine."

"Oh," he said, frowning, "I don't remember that at all."

My husband turned back around to his computer, where he had been working. Afternoon was turning to evening, city crickets and grasshoppers stridulating outside the windows. I shuddered in confusion: this strange inconsonance in the midst of what I thought was perfect understanding. Like a dream that has become a kind of false memory, so unquestionably does it seem to have occurred, I was convinced of a certain assurance: my husband was still "my husband," even at his most pained. I could make a joke and he would "get it." Follow the premise to the conclusion: then he couldn't be dying, no matter how much the pallor of his face reminded me of a dying look.

My father, again. Never mind that my father too seemed to be "my father" the day before he died, though in retrospect I see gestures and looks that were uncharacteristic. Learning against the doorway of our office room, I considered the private memories that come back to me when my husband's sick. I feel selfish that I will my own suffering — or let it in, even if I don't exactly will it — as my husband lies in a deep fog, nauseous, headache imploding.

Nothing reminds two people of how interminable the separation — the metaphysical separation — is between them like pain. As Elaine Scarry famously wrote in *The Body in Pain: The Making and Unmaking of the World*, 1985, "To have pain is to have certainty; to hear about pain is to have doubt." I could try to recount what I know of my husband's pain to create a "picture" of the migraine experience. The truth is, when my husband is sick, he is a question mark. He is an absence. He doesn't have the words to speak of his pain and he doesn't remember very much of it after. When he goes under, as I think of it, he is hurtled down a long corridor, an echo chamber, where pulses and pressure grind him down into a mere bundle of sensation.

And I wonder: how do I live with the pain? I don't mean, how do I adjust to the fact of his migraines, to the sum total of days he spends in bed, to the strict diet that turns us into dour non-wine drinking, anti-aged cheese ascetics. I mean, while he is in pain, how do I exist with him in that pain? The impulse is to empathize. But how can I? I don't have that exact pain. I am blessedly headache-free. Even if I did have headaches, his pain would never *be mine*. And if I try to access my own experience of pain in order to be able to commiserate with him, exist with him in pain, adopt a comportment proper to the hushed, sick-house quiet of the hours when he is out of it, then I self-centeredly subsume his experience into my own.

When my husband is sick, his face recedes from the face I think I know — the beard I have touched as though touching the bark on a tree, full of awe in the sensation of it under my touch, soft and rough both; and the eyes I have discovered so often in half-meditation, pooling around a thought, a view, an emotion.

That face I have kissed, traced, smelled, mapped, excavated, bitten, poked, watched, ignored, followed: suddenly it is gone. It is retracted, figuratively, as when a new face of pain erupts in its place, or literally, when it turns into the pillow, burying into it, to get rid of the light. I have mistaken this alterity for death, doing violence to it, trying to force it into a narrative of suffering I understand — the death of my father — even if it brings me pain to think of my husband in relation to this narrative.

But if my husband — the husband I know, the one who jokes about squirrels we've named Young Sir for their audacious food-stealing, the one who will bury their run-over bodies in the yard so I don't have to see death — is absented, for a time,

am I not brought into communion with his being, the very fact of his existence, so unassailable and beyond my grasp, and so, in a sense, truer than the quotidian him I know? And am I not, then, brought into proximity with the infinite?

To suffer with my husband, then, instead of in him, or in him in me, is to let him go from my grasp into his pain. To let him go into his pain isn't to ignore his suffering or pretend it doesn't exist. It is to commune with his unknowability in those hours of his suffering, to bear witness to his being, laid bare — vulnerable, naked.

———— ❧ ————

When my husband has a migraine, he succumbs in late afternoon, going to bed far earlier than usual and sleeping until late morning. On those nights, I stay up late, sometimes all night, as though to make sure nothing more will touch us or him. I give him quiet, space. I keep the cats occupied. I answer the phone on one ring.

Insomniacs know that the night performs a radical mystery. For every insomniac, there comes a moment, maybe right before the first birds' twittering at dawn, maybe when the last neighbor's light goes out, when the emptiness seems to dilate into infinity. You are, it seems, entirely alone. And yet: not alone. There are countless breathing beings out there, asleep, or so it seems, and you are the only one awake. You must keep vigil.

I keep my husband's space quiet. I keep to another side of the house. But I feel him breathing, feel the distillation of heat, sweat, as I feel the whole of existence rushing into our small house in the deepest hours.

I am called to my husband in his suffering. And when the migraine is ended, I am called to him as a lover, a friend, a partner. Ultimately, the unknowability of him brings us paradoxically closer. I love him all the more because, in the end, I do not know him. I am not him. And he is not me. ❧

"*At the time I wrote this essay, I'd been reading a lot of work by the philosopher Emmanuel Levinas, as well as the Elaine Scarry book that I reference.*"

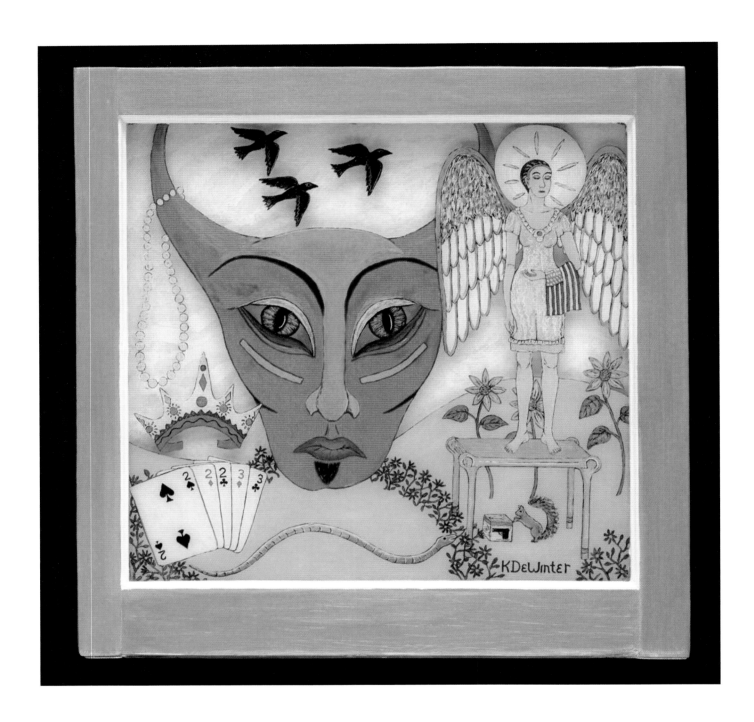

GOOD AND EVIL ©2003 24" by 24"
Karen L. De Winter, Age 60, Seattle, Washington

" 'Good and Evil' is a reverse painting on glass in a wood-framed window with a recessed backboard painting to be seen through the glass. This technique creates depth and shadows. The painting was inspired by the feeling I get when the first inklings of a migraine start. It represents the bright colors of normal life in contrast with the feeling of unease and danger related to the impending headache. "Headache" seems so weak a word in relation to a migraine. Migraines cause you to shut down all your senses, put on dark glasses, lie down, muffle all sounds and ride the waves of pain like some strange and terrible carnival ride. The objects in the painting speak to this dynamic."

Relentless
©2007

Linda Gallant Potts
Age 56, Caledon, Ontario, Canada

A demon lurks within me. It lies in wait, planning the strategy of its next attack. It is merciless, intent on bringing me to my knees.

If I am vigilant, I may feel the signs, the vague discomforts and rumblings that warn me of the danger. Fatigue suddenly overwhelms me. Lights shimmer. Vertigo grabs hold of me and my stomach signals its unrest. In those few frantic moments I erect makeshift barriers and steel myself against the enemy's onslaught. Occasionally, the barricade works: the enemy retreats to his hiding place and rethinks his tactics.

I am rarely so lucky.

"I must move with more stealth," he whispers between clenched teeth. Then he comes by night, when darkness provides subterfuge and sleep relaxes my guard. The shock of pain alters the script of my dreams, turning them to nightmares.

"I will give no time for a defense," he vows, and he arrives like a lightning bolt from within me, a scene reminiscent of an old horror flick. The monster prowls the cage within my skull.

Fury is its fuel. It claws in rage over its captivity and rips at the muscles and ligaments at the base of my neck to escape. Pain attacks there in spasms, making it difficult to keep my head erect. Stiffness spreads to my shoulders, down my back, my arms. If I move I will immediately regret it. My brain bashes inside my skull. The demon travels down my throat and I gag. He lingers in my belly, churning the remnants of my last meal.

His spiny tentacles discover the vulnerability of my temples. They dig at the flesh to escape. The top of my head is slowly being drilled away and I feel the heat of the inflamed vessels within. My ears throb and ring; it pains my eyes to see. Glands in my neck feel full to rupturing. The skin of my face is numb and it hangs, lifeless. I glance in the mirror: the reflection is not me.

My eye sockets, the indented place in front of my ear, my jaw, all threaten to snap. I stretch my mouth wide and feel a slight relief, not enough. My teeth and gums ache as if an over-zealous hygienist has probed and prodded for hours. I want to put my head in a vise, force the bones in my skull back into position.

It has been 18 hours now, and the migraine grows steadily worse. The medicine prescribed for me has not helped; it rarely does. I fight the panic and desperation that will only increase the pain. Instead, I wait it out, knowing full well that this attack could last for days. And like the childhood game of seeing who can go longer without blinking, I am not confident of the outcome. Tonight, my agony convinces me that this time the demon may win. ⮥

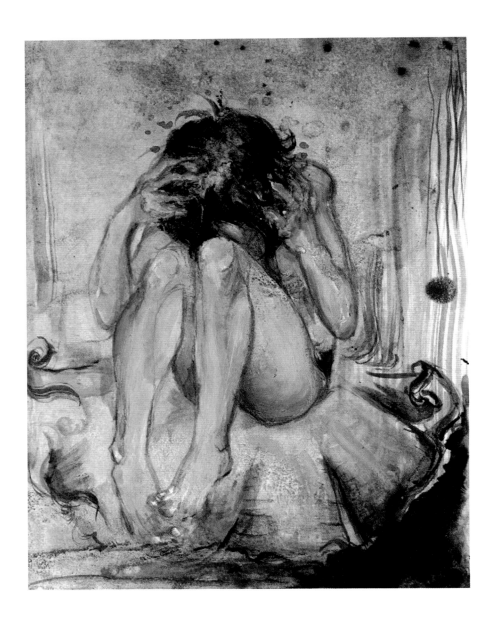

Mygraine
©2007

Donna E. Baxter
Age 52
Sarasota, Florida

Sparklers drowning in pools of moving mercury
obscuring blotches of my vision.
Present despite repeated blinking
in Desperate Denial.
A warning that my body, my HEAD
will no longer belong to me as the
Enemy worms his way into and through
tightening muscles,
winding, crawling up the neck,
inflaming each cell of every tissue.
Blood vessels pumping, throbbing.
Nerve endings on fire and screaming.
Even the hair hurts —
hypersensitive and electric.
The enemy surges forward, upward
into the sinuses and brain matter
settling with a triumphant THUD
behind the left eyeball,
sending throbbing waves in all directions.
Then directly to the GUT,
which churns and burns and demands
equal attention with pounding head trauma.
My enemy.
He promises endless hours of blinding pain,
sleeping on ice,
hopeless efforts to quiet the mind over and
over and over
(what could have triggered this one?)
(what should I take next?)
(what did I do wrong to deserve this?)
(can't I just die?)
(maybe if I move my neck just so)
(maybe if I visualize healing)
and always a tremendous medication hangover.
My enemy.
He keeps his promises
And
his gift is always the same….
the eventual lifting…..relief…..freedom as he
slowly retreats,
my Joy and Gratitude for every single moment that
He is away.

Status Migrainosus

©2006

Heather Nicaise
California

Alone in the dark,
there is a fear of infiniteness.
I hate the pain that envelops me.
I'm afraid it will never end.

There is a fear of infiniteness.
I struggle with the pain.
I'm afraid it will never end.
I cannot see the light.

I struggle with the pain.
Nothing to do but wait.
I cannot see the light
screaming inside my head.

Nothing to do but wait.
The fog, the haze muffles me.
Screaming inside my head,
despair that will remain.

The fog, the haze muffles me.
I pray for its dissolution.
Despair that will remain
until misery releases my soul.

Praying for dissolution—
I hate the pain that envelops me.
The misery releases my soul.

I am alone in the dark.

"I found that the repetitive nature of the pantoum expressed well the nature of migraine disease."

"Status Migrainosus" was originally published on the National Headache Foundation's Web site.

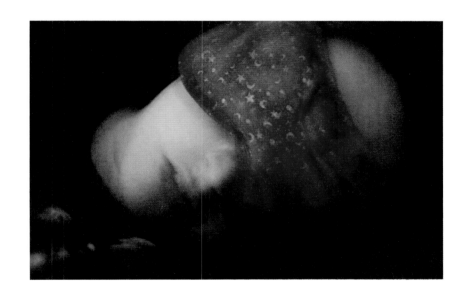

MASK TO BED ©2007
Stacy McKenzie, Age 26, New York, New York

My Migraine Advice:
Don't Listen to Migraine Advice
©2007

Melissa Becker
Age 28
Clearwater, Florida

"I had a migraine once." When I hear those five words, it's a signal to shut my brain off for the next five minutes and nod absently while someone with only the best intentions makes an ass of themselves. If you haven't had the luxury of meeting one of these miracle one-time-only migraine sufferers, here's how their story goes. They had a really bad headache. They take two aspirins and it doesn't go away. Then they take something that says "migraine strength" and it goes away. That's it. I'll have to ask my team of neurologists why we hadn't thought of doing that. Thank you, random person, for giving me that insightful piece of medical advice.

People don't understand that a migraine isn't just a headache. It isn't even a really bad headache. It is your body declaring war on itself with a shock-and-awe attack. The headache is a big part of it but by no means is it the whole thing. There's the dizziness.

The fatigue. The lightshow before your eyes. The feeling of detaching from your body and watching yourself live your life with no control over it. And you can't forget the nauseous feeling that sends you running for the bathroom stall only to kneel there, leaning on the porcelain, debating whether or not something is going to come up. Thank god for wireless laptops because now I can get my work done in there!

I tend to stay at the office during my migraines. If I'm going to feel like there is a slam dancing competition in my cranium, at least I'm going to get paid for it. Besides, the time I tried to follow the advice about lying down in a dark room I was left with nothing to distract me from my thoughts. It might have helped my migraine attack, but it was hard to tell with the panic attack it produced.

I think like most people who have migraines (what should we call ourselves? Migraineies? Migrainanites?) I have my own way of coping with the attacks. It's a complicated ritual involving taking one set of drugs at the first moment signs of an early attack and then keeping an ice pack on my neck. A friend of mine takes a cup of coffee and a nap to stave off hers. What works for one person will probably not work for another, which is why you can tell that the advice dispensers have never really had a migraine. If they did, they'd know that migraines are as unique as children. For those who are new to their migraine, I won't tell you how to fix it. I don't know. Nobody does. But you'll figure it out.

That's the best piece of advice I can give you. Don't think of your migraine as a disease that you will defeat. It isn't. It's more like an obnoxious family member whom you are stuck with until DNA-altering procedures are developed. But just like with any annoying relative, you eventually find a way to co-exist. I am not an optimist by any stretch of the imagination. I don't just think the glass is half-empty, I think that it's not what I ordered in the first place. But if there is a positive lesson from my migraines, it is that they taught me to listen to myself. To be highly attuned to my body's senses and feelings and reactions to the world around me. It was self-awareness, not any prescription or dietary habit, which has allowed me to live with migraines — and to live sometimes without them. ☙

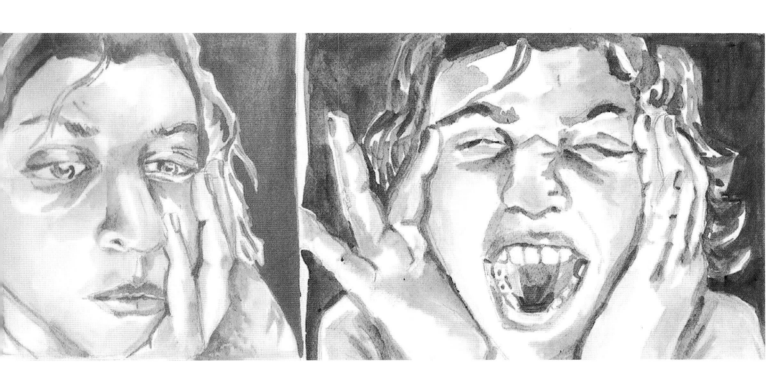

HEADACHE TRIBULATIONS ©2007
Marina Kharkover, Age 22, Little Neck, New York

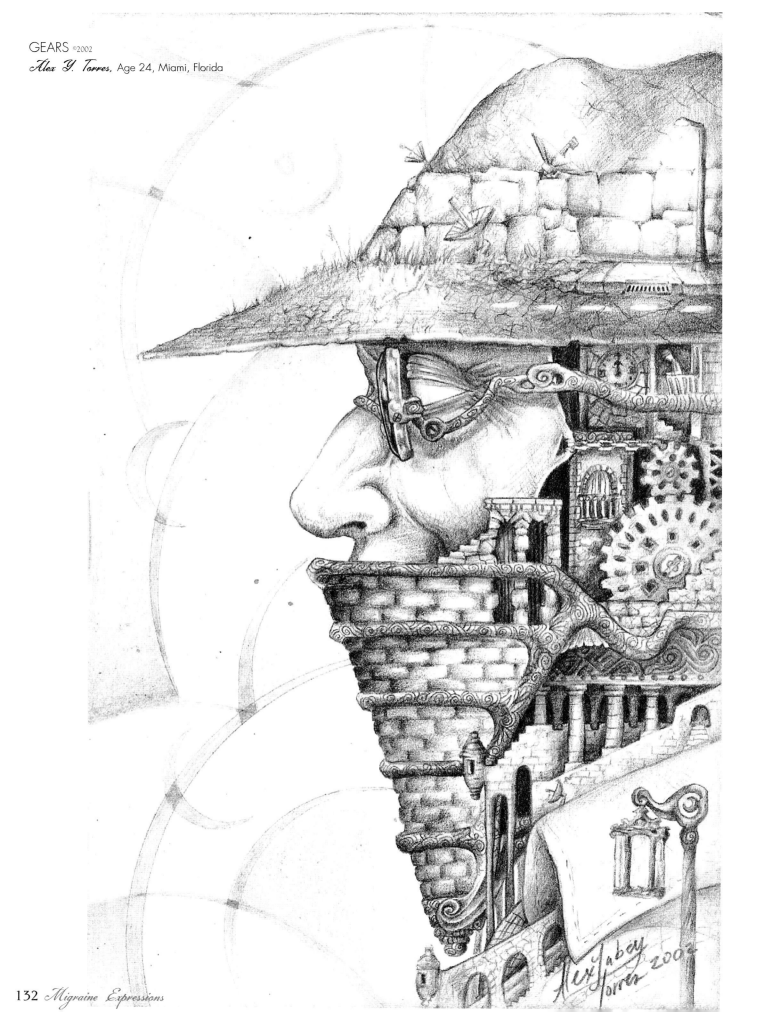

AN UPSIDE TO MIGRAINE PAIN?
The Case for *Hyperthought* ©2007
Michael Gaylor, Age 41, Tidewater, Virginia

When taking inventory of the chronic curses of the human condition, one must of necessity rank near the top the debilitating effects of migraine pain. I am a lifelong migraineur, and my pathology has been so frequent and repressively intense over the years that I am these days resigned to accept it as a normal expression of my physiology. Indeed, most migraineurs are.

After some deep introspection, ironically, much of the time conducted during extreme suffering, I am concerned about such apparent resignation. But, I am increasingly inclined toward and comforted by a belief that there may be something therapeutic and even intellectually enhancing buried deep down in the maelstrom of migraine pain, if I can only figure out how to access it.

Migraine is a paralyzing dysfunction that robs me of appreciable essence of the very thing that defines me as a cognitive being. As an academician, the intellectual dimensions of migraine headache intrigue me to a nearly discombobulated extent. In fact, my preoccupation has become so entrenched that I have actually considered sitting down to quantify the percentage of my life demoted to virtual vegetative stasis by migraine despair. Of course, I have abstained from this depressing exercise, largely on account of the deluge of distress that would inevitably ensue were I to contemplate the measurable degree to which precious snapshots of my sentience have been absconded by the specter of migraine. But I cannot deny my sore temptation.

After what feels like an eternity of migraine, I now view the condition as tantamount to "living loss of life." I believe that any veteran migraineur will appreciate the aptness of this phrase as it poignantly describes the familiar desperation and austerity of recurring periods of life without the ability to live. Viewed in this way, it can be emotionally calamitous to consider the loss of what we already know to be precarious, particularly when intermittent misery of such power is averaged over a lifetime. But, curiously enough, this condition appears to have spawned in me a new and sometimes extraordinary feeling of elevated cognitive ability.

Migraine pain is sinister and debilitating. Indeed, the very nature of the disorder renders mental and physical activity intolerable. Yet, paradoxically, it also intimates a curious upside for me in that strange flashes of intensely creative and analytical thought now often accompany my attacks. It's as if the sheer magnitude of my pain transforms my psyche into a kind of altered state of consciousness. I know not what else to call it. Because I am one who likes to assign or pigeonhole things and phenomena into conceptual strata in my mind for the loftier purposes of understanding, I have designated this peculiar state of being as *hyperthought*. This vexing circumstance might best be likened to the effect produced by ingesting a psychoactive drug. In addition to being just plain fascinating, it has, on so many levels, redefined the total migraine headache experience for me.

Though hyperthought is intellectually engrossing, it is also quite the conundrum in that it is not generally a pleasant or utilitarian or natural physiological state. I do not think, for instance, that it will enable me to address the more pressing ostensible problems of everyday cognitive life.

Thus, I would not recommend migraine pain as a prescription for the doldrums of daily living, or as a tonic to heal writer's block or the like. But, during what are typically Herculean efforts to focus my tattered mind away from the clutches of throbbing pain toward higher planes of therapeutic escape, it is evident that I am able to attain a bizarre clarity of thought that is not otherwise possible.

There is something almost metaphysical about hyperthought. Nevertheless, it is demonstrably there and even potentially medicinal, if only detectably. As such, I think it could be a salient point of focus during migraine attack that may actually promote healing. Of course, recognizing this in the abstract is easy. The real difficulty lies in devising a strategy for manipulating this heightened awareness for rational productivity and therapeutic remediation. As you might imagine, this is proving to be another matter of applied determination entirely. The concomitant stew of headache trauma presents formidable mental and even physical challenges. But, as a migraineur who has until now largely been unable to fathom even a glimpse of redeeming value in this affliction, I have summarily committed to meeting this challenge head-on and pressing forward into this uncharted, and hopefully eventually practical, realm of hyperthought.

In the meantime, my crude attempts to exploit this weird mental circumstance for tangible cognitive and therapeutic gain have actually begun to bear some fruit. With each migraine bout I become more convinced that I am on to something strangely and innately positive disguised deep down within the cavernous anguish of migraine pain. As an example, on more than one occasion, when I am visited by hyperthought during a migraine attack, I have achieved what I believe are perceptible degrees of deeper rumination about myriad things. I do not deny that I encounter much difficulty discerning anything with any great precision within the sharply brilliant opacity of migraine pain. Yet, this degree of musing provides a mysterious comfort that seems in some instances to almost literally take me by the hand and guide me through the murky vortex of migraine delirium. The result has been realization of a modicum of enlightened thought seemingly possessing some therapeutic value.

Upon what I meditate during hyperthought can be decidedly random and unpredictable and will usually span a gamut from the relatively existential, such as the meaning of life and the origins of space and time to the relatively mundane, such as what I will eat when the wretchedness subsides and why my cats have "pooches." In fact, I have found that the extremity of the mundane will sometimes be sufficient to quell my pain, even if only perceptibly. Accordingly, in as much as possible under this kind of totalitarian duress, I will often choose to purposefully obsess on the mundanity in hopes of achieving an analgesic effect. So, it appears then that I have progressed toward some meaningful recognition of an enigmatic upside to migraine pain amidst some rather foreboding odds and in so doing have made strides in regulating my disease toward at least a semblance of cognitive self-improvement.

I am painfully aware that, to the casual reader, and even to fellow migraineurs, my vision of hyperthought as a potentially benevolent byproduct of this chronic disease may at first smack of grandiose wishful thinking and even downright delusion born of a life of suffering. Perhaps this is so. Who knows? I have certainly been accused of being weird by many and with some regularity throughout my lifetime. One thing is quite clear, though. The magnificent scope and processes of the human mind are infinitely convoluted and may never be fully comprehended. Thus, at this embryonic point in our evolution, we simply cannot know such things with any real confidence.

However, veteran migraineurs do know one thing better than anyone else. During the gripping incendiary discomfort of migraine attack, one will joyously reach for any and all remedies real or imagined that promise even meager relief. Moreover, given the power of migraine to pilfer cognition and perturb physical harmony, I think any reasonable person would agree that hyperthought should be considered a potentially positive aspect of this disease worthy of concentration and further examination. Indeed, in my perennial search for enlightenment, and more simply as a practical matter of discovering new mechanisms of coping and healing, I now embrace this view and condition with new vigor and expend every effort to formally enter and explore hyperthought each and every time I am assaulted by migraine headache pain. ☙

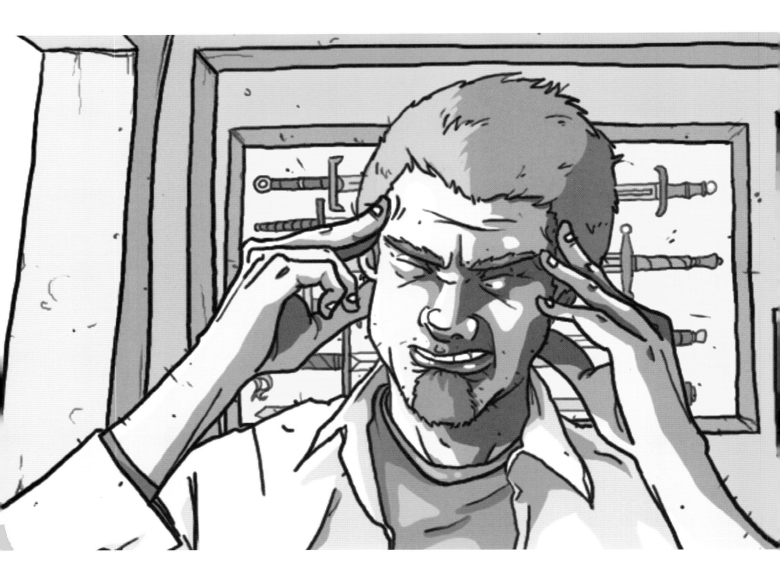

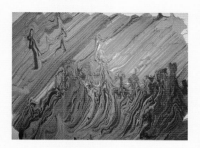

THE SUMMONING

rant   rant   rant   displace anger
    rant   rant   eyes of eyes in sockets not depth
    rant   fingers of bone beneath asphalt
    anger   anger displaced
    fear in the thriving inept
    not eyes not
    tongues not eye
    teeth not eyes
    iris not eye iris no
    not I
    athena crushing my cornea
    throbbing inside   pressure
    jackhammer
    release
    release not I
    not eye
    feathers
    glue   too close
    sunfall
    drown
    fear father in debt
    eyes without sight
    light draws shadow
    hide in a black room
    hide in a black room
    think about light
    anger
        displace anger
    rage   RAGE   RAGE   RAGE RAGE
    wet rage
    sockets not eyes
    see without thinking
    fingers
    blind touch   displace
    eyes
    hide eyes in a jar

Art & poem by *Ken Sleight,* ©2007
Age 32, Lansing, Michigan

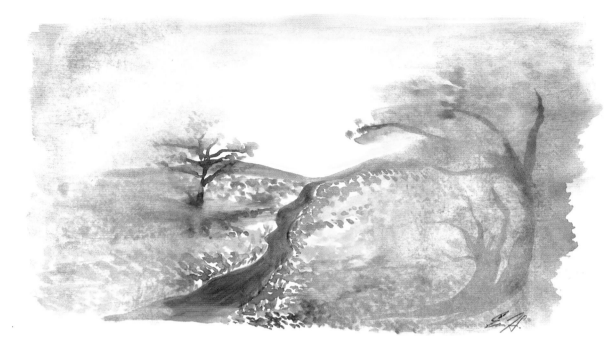

BLURRY VISION ©2007

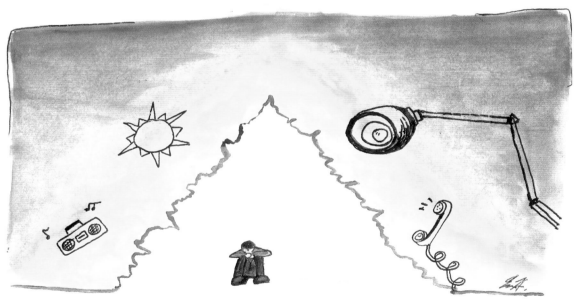

NOISE AND LIGHT ©2007

Evan Hilsenberg, Age 23, Seattle, Washington

"My mom has suffered from migraines for as long as I can remember, these paintings reflect both the "blurry side vision" she says she experiences at the onset of a migraine and the impact of noise and light when she begins to get a headache."

My Migraines
©2007

Michele D. Solano
Age 30
Renton, Washington

Tiny white spots,
As if someone takes a picture too close,
You blink and pray they'll go away.

Pressure behind your eyes,
As if someone is squeezing your brain,
And you begin to stumble and sway.

Instant pain,
As if a sledgehammer just hit you,
Right in the middle of your forehead.

Nausea from hell,
As if you've ingested poison;
Making you wish that you were dead.

Sight and sound
Are your instant enemies;
You crave a room filled with silent black.

Prayers and tears
Are all you can manage,
Begging someone to take the pain back.

Seconds from hours,
You can't tell the difference;
You just hold on until it's done.

Relief and exhaustion
Are the final stage,
As you hope this will be the last one.

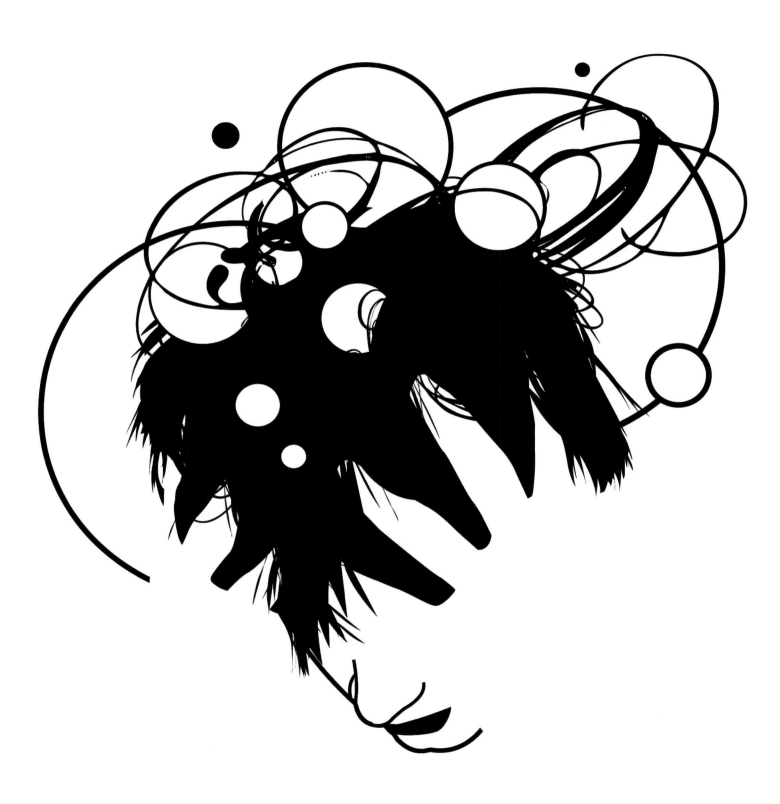

Cherry Tree Headache
©2007

Jaya Hobbs
Age 36
Jamaica Plain, Massachusetts

monster moments lapse into the wind
and get caught in
and wrapped around
a branch of the cherry tree
out my window i feel the stillness
of a four thirty in the morning yoga pose
that, too, gets caught
and wrapped around

(my eyes, bloodshot like these summer cherries,
lose vision to the blackest of autumn crows)

like tangled black hair wrestling a mess
the cherry tree has its branches
with so much of my life caught and wrapped around it
with so much of my headspin twirl

The Lump of Coal
©2007

Grace K. Rajendran
Seattle, Washington

Ten thousand tons of fury
Pressure, that breaks
More than a few
But this is your life
And all this agony, nothing new

Somehow you find the strength
When others crack under the strain
You seem to find the strength
Despite the mind-rending pain

Nature chooses well
Her survivors, steadfast
And True Blue
Others surrender and fall
But that shall never be you

A mere lump of coal
Soon learns to yield, learns to give
But the hardest stone
Inflexible
Will never live

So rest your weary self
Soothe your tired soul
And know that here stands a diamond
Where once there was coal

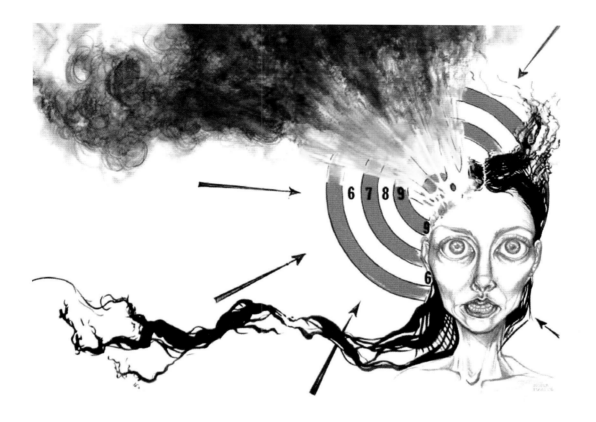

Migraine and Life ©2007

When deep in the throes
of an unrelenting migraine
one naturally wonders
how this excruciating pain
could possibly be
compatible with life

Migraine Woman ©2007

you can recognize her easily,
She must wear dark glasses to block out sunlight,
dark, loose clothing to hide her bloated belly,
loose hair since tight up do's will just not do,
an NTI dental device to keep her jaw unclenched,
ear plugs to block out irritating noises,
a breathe easy strip on her nose to help
her breathe easy,
an ice pack head band and neck band,
a pill box ring to always be prepared,
a medic alert bracelet for emergency trips,
Have You Seen Her?

Both poems by
Teresa Cantilli Ramos
Age 46, Garden City South, New York

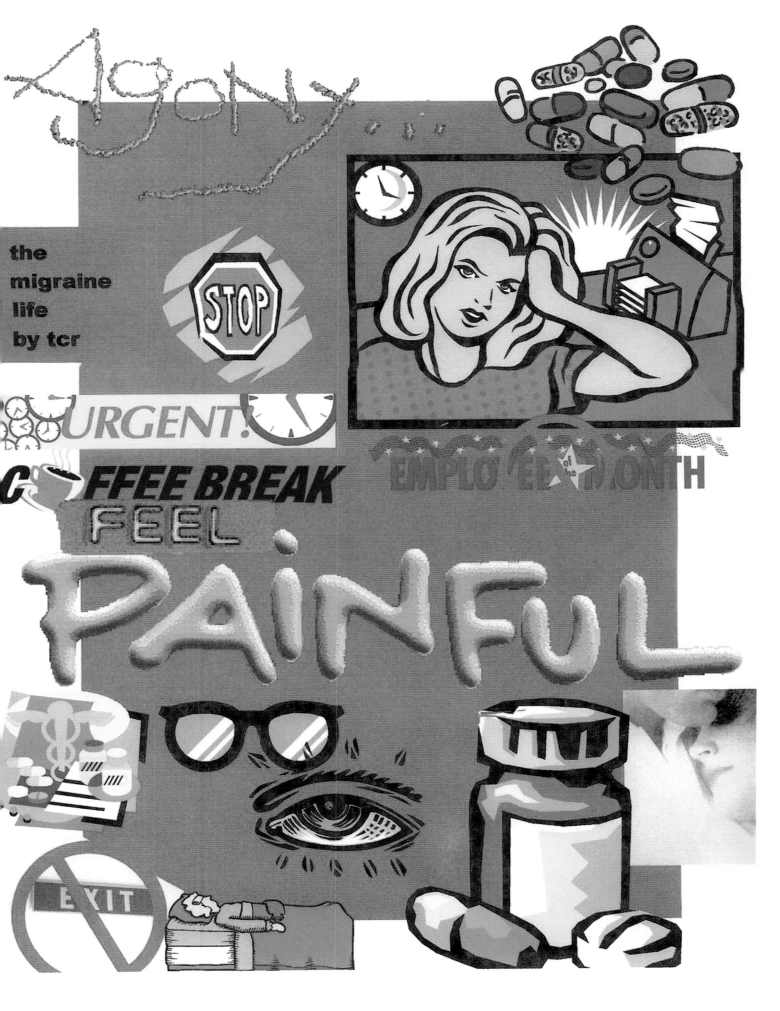

Millie Simon-Dufault, RN
© 2007
Age 48
Litchfield, New Hampshire

What is it about a migraine's laser piercing pain that sends me into a light show of creative ideas? I've never researched this phenomenon, so I have no idea if my fellow sufferers share the weirdness.

My head feels like it's about to explode, but the HGTV addict in me is bounding through the home decorating department at a frantic pace.

"Oh My God! The graphics on these pillows are perfect."

Pain pulses like neon, but I massage my temples and press on.

Oooh. I grab the comforter. Last one. "Look at the quality. Tight weave, organic fabric, that baby won't pill...and it blends with the pillows..."

I toss the pillows on top and confirm my choice. The pain intensifies, but the 600 count sheet sets on sale catch my eye.

"Bold with just the right punch of color for the room."

I really should drop my head onto that satiny pillow case right about now, but who can resist the heart pounding excitement. The artistic juices flow like lava while my head erupts like a volcano.

Squeezing my eyes shut against the fluorescent lights, I rub my head and bargain with myself.

Just one more aisle, I promise. "Oh, faux suede blankets."

A tactile girl, I feel the luxurious nap.

"Oh yeah. That'll work."

My stomach flutters with anticipation of my new bedroom. Or maybe it's the nausea starting. I better go faster.

"Brushed nickel lamps. Sophisticated, especially against a chocolate brown wall, metropolitan..." Where's the paint?

Why do stores play the music so darn loud, anyway? Haven't they ever heard of easy listening, or silence, for that matter? I can't take any more! Black frames, a couple of abstract pieces. Okay, done.

Amazing! The bedroom makeover I put off for months comes together in the span of 30 minutes thanks to the lightning bolts knifing through one side of my brain.

The drive home is a little scary, with the blurred vision and all. I think a bomb is going off in my head. It's a war zone up there. My ears are ringing.

"Oh My God. I have the best idea for a book. A thriller. The plot twists and turns burst through my brain like fireworks, one after another."

Finally, I'm home. Where's my bed? Maybe I'll save the novel for the next migraine. ➣

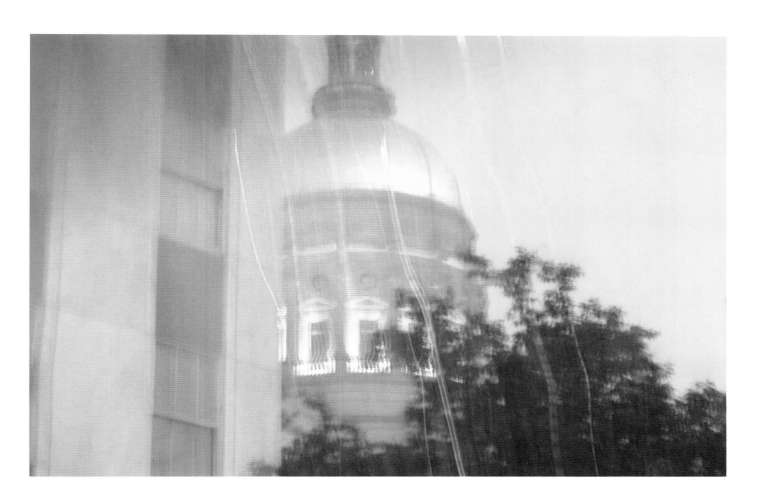

MY WORLD THROUGH THE EYES OF A MIGRAINE ©2007
Vanessa Neely, Age 52, Newnan, Georgia

"During migraine days, life more often than not becomes a blur. This photograph depicts how I see things when suffering with migraine pain."

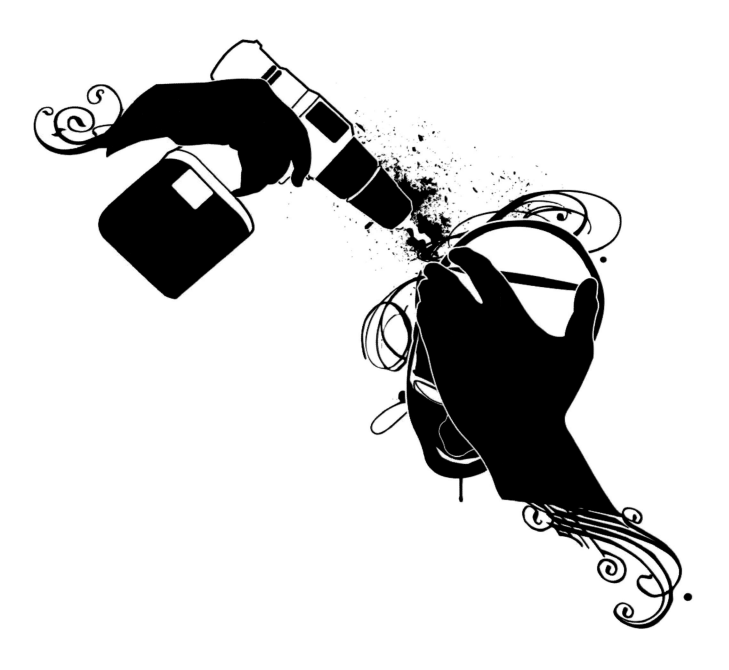

Spinning Out of Control

©2007

Bernadette Garzarelli
Age 55
Beach Haven, New Jersey

Held captive by voices in my head
Take the pills, no don't take the pills
It's dark and painful in this place
Falling deeper into the abyss
No light in sight

The drill continues to penetrate
Go ahead and take the pills
Sleep doesn't come easily
A desperate thought returns
Take the whole bottle
What do I have to lose

Family and friends who love me
Try to empathize and keep me alive
What do they know, they can't feel my pain
Only words of encouragement not to give up

Another day, another month, another year
Knowing somewhere deep inside
Life is worth living, where's the sun
Ah, I just caught a glimpse

Fighting the Flood
©2007

A quiet silent drip
Ignoring the warning of what's to come
Not today
I'm pushing on.

Droplets become a pool
And I am barely treading water
Take a breath
I'm pushing on.

Building up around me
Pulling me farther from the shore
Don't lose sight
I'm pushing on.

Rough water batters me
Being slowly crushed beneath the flood
Just let go
I'm sinking down.

Searching for a warm light
I'm cradled, rolling on each passing wave
Find relief
I will push on.

Lauren Koblara
Age 26
West Brookfield, Massachusetts

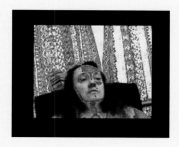

©2007 *Sande R. Waybill*, Age 41, Wollongong, NSW, Australia

Attack!
©2005

Ice assaults my cheek,
Slowly, too slowly,
I recognise the warning sign,
The numbness I feel kick-starts my reaction,
But too late to halt my decline.

The enemy within is en route,
Intentions are definitely hostile,
Borg-like the pain invades,
Resistance is futile.

But once again, I engage my opponent,
Chemical warfare is still my weapon of choice,
Inevitably the conflict escalates,
Forced to retreat, I adopt the fallback position: the coffin,
Silent and still, darkness dominates.

Hours later, the siege is over,
Battle weary, knowing that victory is always short-lived,
My old foe will never be defeated as I wish,
It is merely latent, awaiting opportunity,
A lifelong condition to be managed, not vanquished.

Ellen Williams
Worcestershire, England

*"I wrote this poem at a time when I was experiencing very frequent migraines —
the war theme was an attempt to express how embattled I felt."*

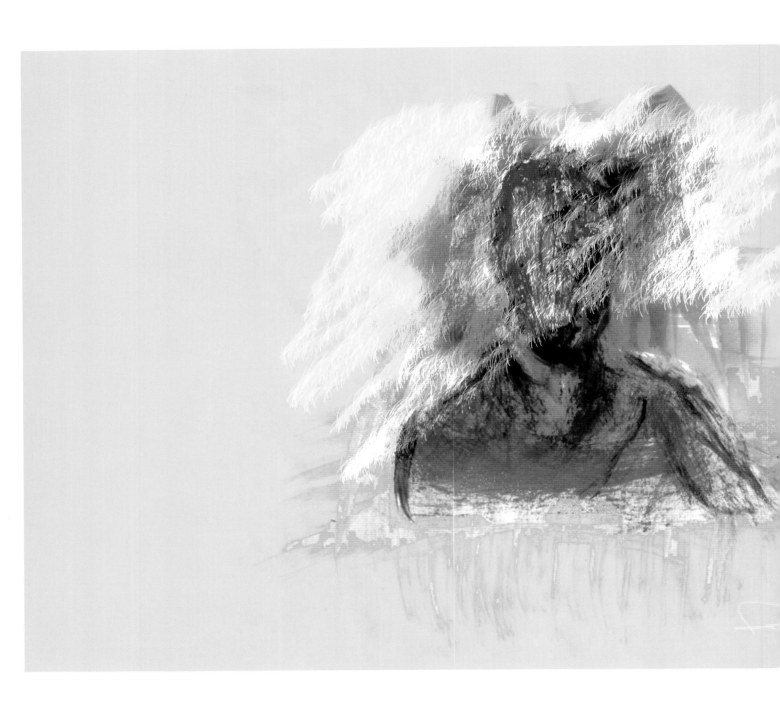

it's a yellow, sick sort of nausea,
the kind you get from riding in cars on a hot bright day
it lies at the back and bottom of everything else.
the blind spots sort of like when you've been looking at the sun
except they shimmer sickeningly, then dissipate, leaving in their wake
a leaden thumb that presses relentlessly on a certain spot in the top
left quarter of the skull, as the rest of the fingers mash together the
throbbing remains of what lies under there.

the changing barometer always brings it.
a capsule a day gives a laughable pretense of control, in reality only
reining back the angry rising murmur, increasing silently day to day
until it finally overcomes and surges free.

Jessica Oei ©2004
Age 26, Cambridge, Massachusetts

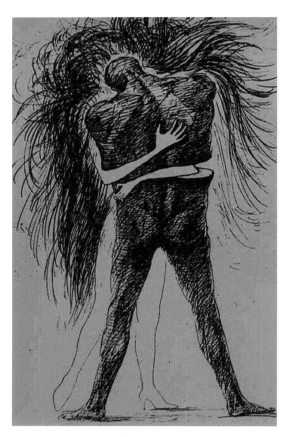

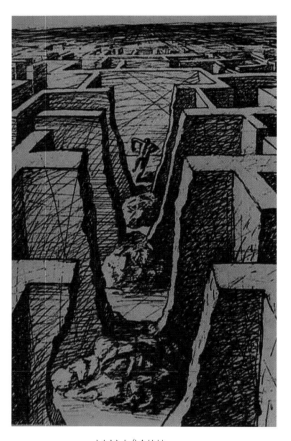

MAN/WOMAN ©2007
*The enemy within, a migraine, taking over myself
and my judgment.*

MAN/WALL ©2007
*Running man, hitting wall after wall, continuous pain and
challenge – no end in sight.*

Louise Donovan, Age 46, Lower Bucks County, Pennsylvania

The Migraine ©2007

I am a congestion, a collision. I am an inflammation.
I am tension and toxins and tightness.
I am the heavy-binded, small-minded interior other;
I am a hostile predator.

Alexandra E. Dickerman
Marin, California

The Harrowing Climb ©2007

The ascension begins.
Walking, pacing up the rugged hill.
Racing hearts with nervous nauseous prophesies.
Faster, rising above the skyline,
Thinning air quickens the dizziness.
Flashing specks of light grow more intense with every blink.
Steeper, scaling the sharp point of rock, jolting out of the jagged wall,
Pressure paralyzes thinking,
Mounting to the very top, with blinding pain
Stretching me from each end
And jointly pressing me within myself, thumping.

I've made it through this struggle for now.
The dark, comforting descent brings a temporary release,
I must prepare for the next climb.

Lynann Butkiewicz
Age 24, Brooklyn, New York

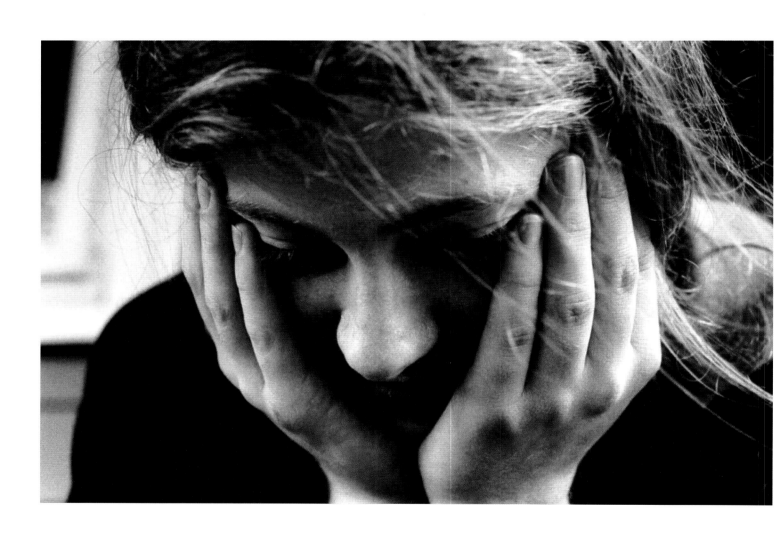

GRAY DAY ©2007

Robin Kuniski, Age 31, Halifax, Nova Scotia, Canada

Party Crasher
©2007

Michelle Euza
Age 33
Miami, Florida

The music's going and I'm dressing up...
tonight I'm going to be social.
Friends in from out of town and I'm feeling great.
The doorbell rings and I leap so fast for that knob
-STRIKE-
I've been attacked.
Inform friends, I cannot make it after all.

Why oh why do you sneak up on me?
We were having such a great day,
you were asleep and I was awake,
Living.
I'm young and deserve some fun! Why must I go lie down now
with a wet towel over my head. Why must I sit in the dark alone,
Why must I wonder why.

I'll cease the moment, but I am not stripping.
You have not defeated me. This dress stays on,
these shoes remain.

An hour later, you're extinct.
I don't know where you've disappeared to.
I don't care. I'm calling a taxi,
Because I'm outta here!!

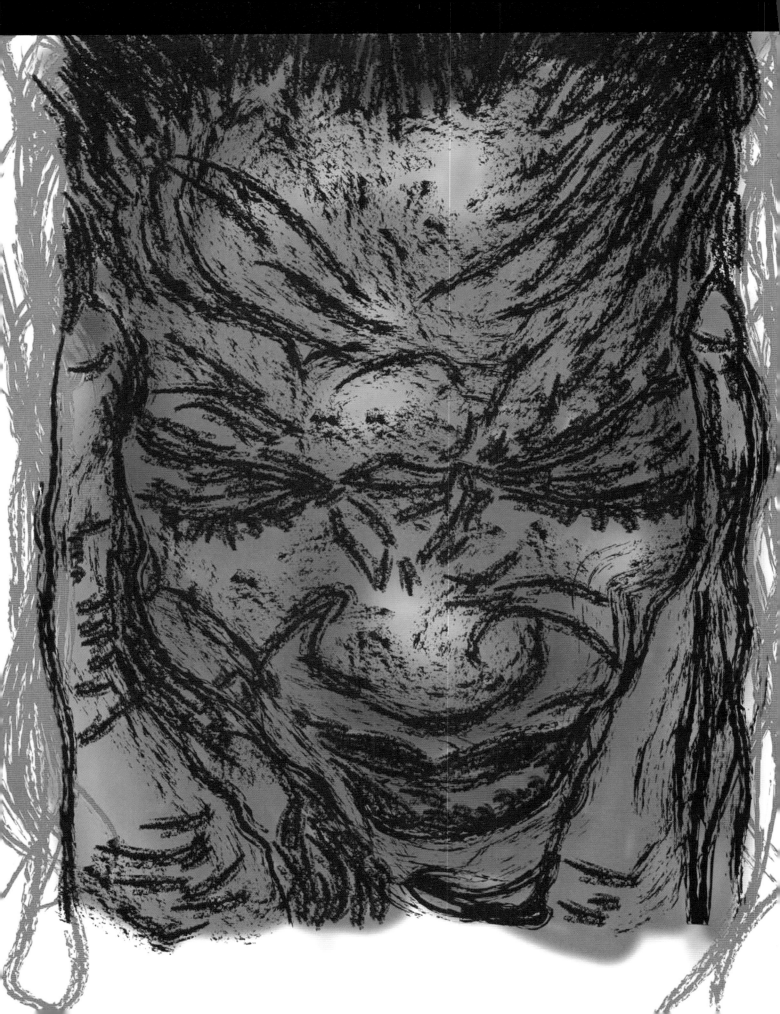

(MY)graine story ©2007

I have suffered from migraine headaches since I was in my teens. If you had asked me when I was younger to rate my pain, I would have said an eight or a nine. The importance of subjective comparisons is not lost on me.

I try to express in words to others the agony I feel during my migraine attacks. You would be amazed at how few people have been shaken by the shoulders violently, or have hit their head on the corner of a cabinet at full human speed. There are no words. I do not require pity for my condition, only understanding. I am reminded of a co-worker who said to me with a slight smile, "I am so stressed out I have given myself a migraine," and I thought to myself, "Look at you all upright and forming complete sentences. I would love to have your migraines."

Please do not trivialize migraines, please do not use them as an excuse to miss work and take a day to sleep late; I would never dream of calling in sick faking oozing pustules simply to watch my favorite soap opera in real time. When I have a migraine attack, I cannot function. It is not a choice and it is not a headache. That being said it is also not any more debilitating than say, diabetes. I have to pay attention to my eating and sleeping habits and my stress levels; I still get migraines, but I can take control of my illness and reduce my risk of attack, and I do.

In the past few years my migraines have evolved into cluster headaches, at least that is what I am told is the cause for the gerbil trying to gnaw his way out of my brain from the core. I have named my gerbil Athena, in tribute to the myth of the goddess's birth from the head of Zeus. As I writhe in pain, I use that particular myth as a distraction and take comfort in the idea that Zeus can sympathize with my pain. I suffer the pain of the gods, and I survive, I excel — and I am grateful for every pain-free moment.

Artwork and essay by
Tifni Richards
Portland, Oregon

STORYLAND ©2007

Patri Collins, Age 41, Seattle, Washington

my wife Gila's world flipped in the detergent aisle of Target one Sunday afternoon about six months ago. She called me at home where I was playing trains with our two-year old son, Urban. Gila's voice was amazingly calm considering how she thought she was losing her sight. I mused that it might be the store's fluorescent lights or that she had been to the gym and hadn't eaten in a while.

"Maybe," Gila said but I could tell by her tone that something else was up.

We met at the emergency room an hour later. I have no idea how she managed to drive there and didn't ask.

Gila hadn't suffered any more sight loss, the world had leveled out to be fuzzy and only occasionally upside down. She stared into a dirty aquarium in the corner of the waiting room while taking her place amongst a motley collection of Sunday afternoon gardening accidents, panic attacks, and confusion. A pair of clown fish darted around in the aquarium's dank water. Gila said that looking at the fish was the only thing that kept her from feeling nauseous. Her place in line to see the doctor kept getting pushed back by what the emergency room nurse called "bleeders." The waiting minutes felt like hours, at times I was convinced Gila was going to die.

There was a point in our life when everyone we met had a rat story. We were battling an unwelcome visitor in our Seattle apartment. All I had to do was mention the little critter and the usually tacit Seattle native would chime in with his or her rat experience. Neighbors opened up to me, co-workers embraced me, even tight-lipped bus riders let loose on how they dealt with the rats of their lives. After several near-comical run-ins with the rat in our apartment, and finally finishing it off in a not-so-funny fashion, Gila and I crafted our own rat story, ready to add to the tome of solidarity in the human vs. rat saga.

The wait in the emergency room doubled for Urban and me when Gila was finally called in to see a doctor. Urban's patience had long run thin, while his dinner time had been neglected. I fed him trail mix from the vending machine, then distracted him with wheelchair races down an empty hospital corridor. Urban kept asking where "Mama" was. I tried to explain to him what was wrong even though I didn't know. Two year-olds like to get answers. When they don't they tend to ask more questions.

By the time the second rat entered our lives, Urban had been born. By that time we found out that people's rat stories paled to their pregnancy/delivery stories. Once again, the stories rained upon on us from predictable and unsuspecting sources the moment Gila made a public appearance with her extended belly. From the adventures relayed to us it was amazing that the human race had made it out of the first millennium. Within a few short months we too had a birth story that was neither unique nor bizarre but somehow incredible.

I let Urban win the wheelchair races, which only temporarily got him off the scent that there was something wrong with his Mama. Sensing a meltdown in that hospital corridor, I pulled out the big guns in the form of a packet of M&Ms from the vending machine. Awake past his bedtime, far from home, and eating chocolate was about as good as it got for Urban. He didn't ask about his Mama anymore, which didn't mean that I stopped worrying about her.

Although uncommon, it seemed like we knew a lot of people who had brain aneurysms. The stories were ghastly, details horrific, yet the survival rate was promising. For some friends it was a small scar on the back of the head easily concealed by hair; for others a radical change in lifestyle, complete with constant monitoring and medication. A friend had just returned from living in Iceland where she told me how the government was encouraging immigration in hopes of diversifying the island's gene pool that carried a propensity for brain clots in teenagers. There's something about abandoned hospital corridors on Sunday nights that allowed me to remember every brain aneurysm story I had ever heard and fear if Gila and I would soon be crafting one of our own.

Gila finally returned to the waiting room. The diagnosis was a migraine. The doctor was positive of this, no aneurysm, pregnancy, or anything to do with a rodent. The migraine was the first of Gila's life. The doctor practically promised that there would be more. The hospital pharmacy dispensed some pills that didn't do anything. We all went home in the same car finding that we were already recounting migraine stories we had heard.

Somehow, this made her migraine a little better. Not much, but a bit. Two days in bed with the lights off helped too. More than the stories. Gila was back at work by Wednesday. By that time the stories really began to flow. Family members came forth like they were revealing long-kept secrets. Friends recounted migraine experiences with the intensity of soldiers returning from war. There were stories of teenage years lost to the migraines, relationships that suffered, and opportunities lost. One friend got a migraine whenever she drank orange juice. Another friend had recently turned vegan in hopes of keeping her weekly attacks at bay.

Again, we felt like we had been admitted to a secret society with the experience, initiated with arcane stories. Luckily, there's only been one migraine since that first. Rats have also stayed out of our lives, Urban probably won't be getting a sibling anytime soon, and no one we know has had a brain aneurysm as of late. Perhaps there was a catharsis in telling the stories. ❧

Migraine Is Real

©2007

Marjorie Farrington
Age 50
Canton, North Carolina

Migraine pain, I could say it's like my shadow
But a shadow is behind you and disappears
in the dark
I could say it's like your own reflection
But your reflection is in front of you,
something clearly seen
the migraine is inside, pain defines me,
something you can't see
To others it's as if it can't be seen,
it's not real
To me, it's become who and what I am,
everything I feel
I could say migraine is my life,
But a life is something that you live
Migraine has taken away my life,
A life I don't remember
what it feels like to live,
To have it back, oh what I would give.
I hold to hope and pray for
relief from this pain
It's like living through
a drought with no sign of rain
It's crying for help and
your words are ignored
It's being looked at like you're crazy,
looking for an excuse
for attention or that you're just lazy
When the pain is lower and you're grateful for relief
Just when you think you can start to live again
Pain is back full force, no life you know,
taken, migraine takes it
like a thief
I pray to God again for relief
while I still can
soon pain will be all that I will be,
Pain no one will believe
because it's something they can't see

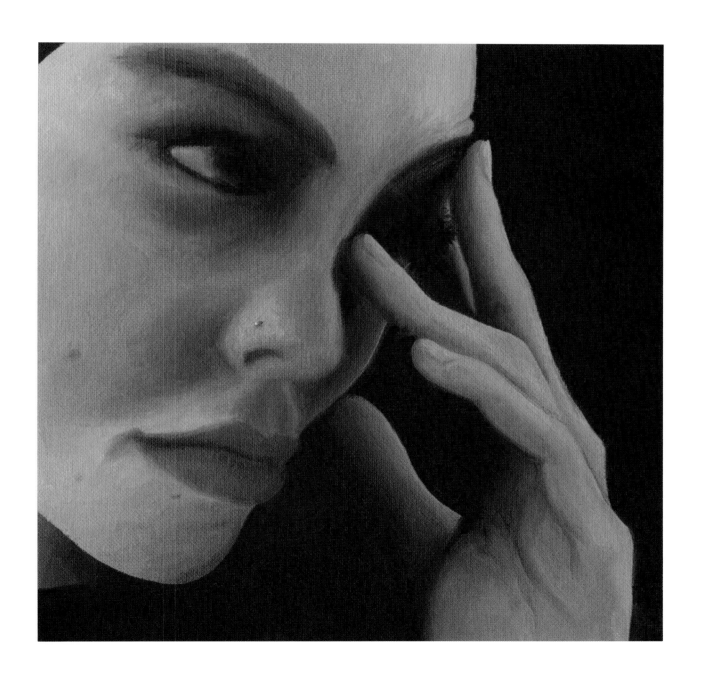

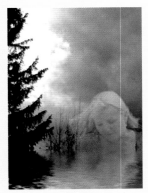

Zoë's Migraine ©2007

Migraines and the Forces of Nature
©2007

Pounding
Blasts akin to thunder and lightning
Splitting
Lighting strikes terminate with intense force
Throbbing
Water courses through tight canyon walls
Wobbling
Blurry outline looms upon the distant horizon
Dizzying
Blasts of light cut like a laser through the water
Nauseating
Swirling bitter liquid envelops the helpless landscape
Irritating
Swarms of egocentric molecules bombard the atmosphere
Devastating
Another forest fire hungrily consumes the innocent trees
Silencing
Electricity ceases and quiets the roiling waves

Zoë Marlowe
Age 48
Logan, Utah

"Migraines are difficult for anyone, but creating art from the suffering seems to help shape the pain into a different perspective."

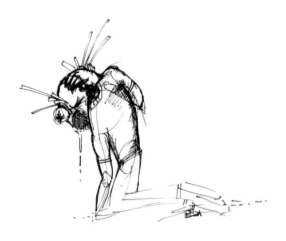

Scott Bennett ©2007

Hello, Brain? Meet Skull
©2007

Last night sleep came. This morning, a red bastard. A beast populating the skull's side. Skulking its way from neck base — that mark from years past still there to decide what will halt and what will pass — then lingering as any familiar friend would, straining in a spot that cannot be reached with pressing, frantic fingertips. Behind the ear it oscillates, radiating crimson no doubt, limbs nimbly reaching luxuriously as its trunk grows up with a strength fed by nightmares, grinding molars, paranoia. Until, finally, I'm awake, dumbed-down, thinking a satin-covered pillow should provide support. Curled like a hedgehog withdrawing into herself, sweat clings above my lip. He searches, rubs the temple radiating undulations like an amplifier, in and out, noticeable and throbbing. Eyes shut tightly I search for somnolence to sink into, channel peppermint and crisp air. This distortion might be soothed sneakily but honestly, by sheer will and the desire for a good day.

Elizabeth Weiss McGolerick
Maryland

Phantom Tango ©2007

the beat is faint, the dance slow
    so slow I'm not sure we're dancing
my partner is but a shadow
    waiting to become more than a phantom

the disco ball that so blithely
    cast shards of light upon my eyes
forecast my partner's arrival
    yet I had dared hope he would not follow

but the beat strengthens
    and the dance intensifies
the steps we've danced before
    are too familiar and unmitigatedly unwelcome

we turn and dip, this direction then that
    an intimate tango
with each dip, my stomach rebels
    the dips so deep my head ricochets off the floor

he shows no pity
    but dances the dance his sadistic way
and when I am beyond spent, he departs
    without so much as a bow at the end

Migraine is a merciless partner
    a relentless partner
a murderess I would gladly become
    if only I could slay him

Teri Robert
Age 53, Washington, West Virginia

Melon Head ©2007

IT begins.
The body in the bed.
Vine-like tendrils swirl up my neck,
Wrapping me neatly, harshly,
As Gulliver in Lilliput.
The bedroom fades....
I am grey-dry growth in a yellow-brown field.
Anaconda vines snap and surge,
as a nova star explodes.
Gargoyle pain pops my skull.
I AM MELON HEAD.
My self... no more
This ripe melon grows, and creaks, and splits.
Scattered seeds of thought lie useless in the now arid air.

Gloriana Casey
Altadena, California

"For me, a migraine is best described by Shakespeare's Hamlet,
'...the undiscovered country...' ."

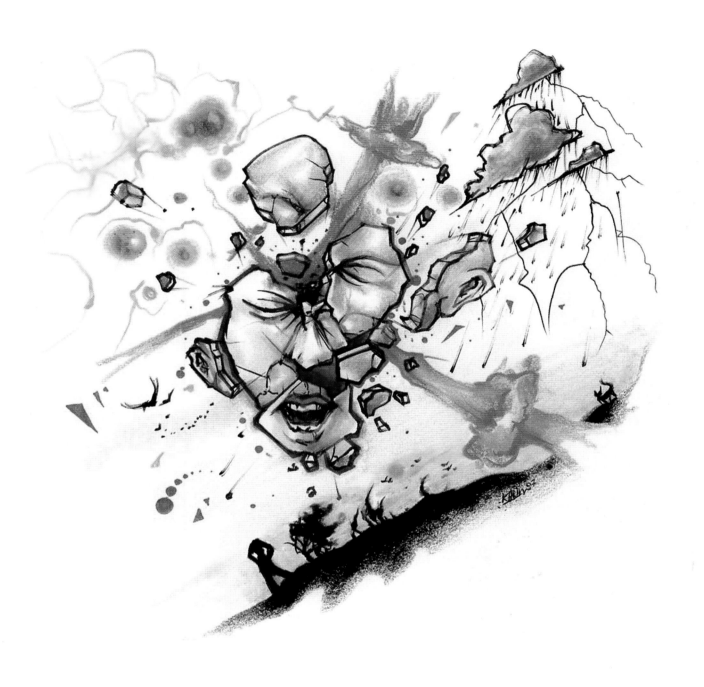

©2007 Ink, Pen, and Crayon

Karim Hetherington, Age 27, Birmingham, United Kingdom

"This piece depicts a shattered head with explosions breaking it like rock, and flashing lights; I experience this when I get a migraine. But there is hope in the picture, as the sun is still there."

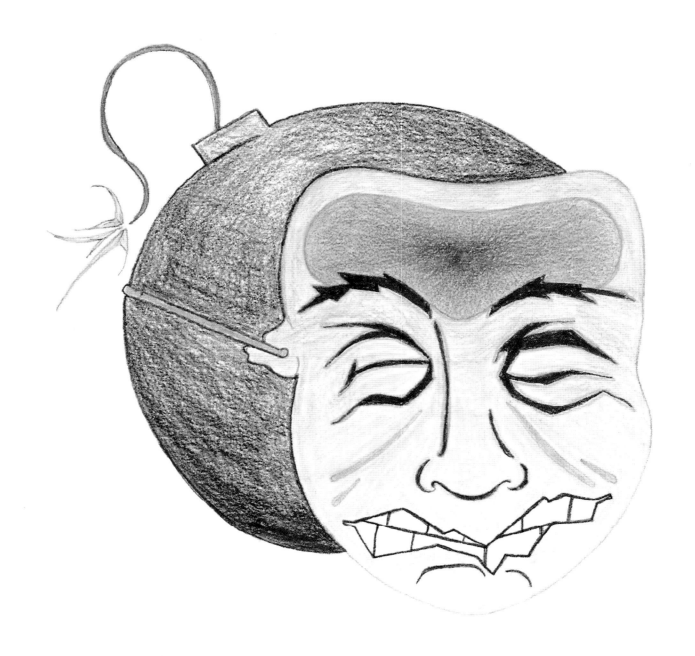

Migraine Analogies
©2007

A scream within my head.
My surroundings disappear as my concentration centers on the area above my eyes.
Pressure continues to build.
Warning signs, then it finally materializes.
A volcano without eruption.
A thunderstorm without lightning.
Until it finally disappears just like all the seconds of the day.

Art and poem by
Rima Rahal
Age 20

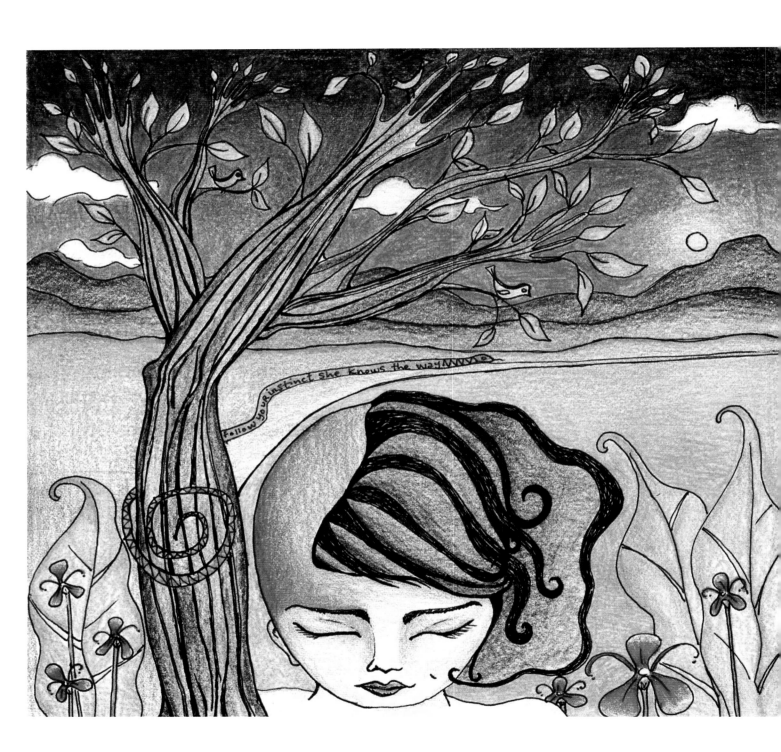

Michelle Melin-Rogovin

Living with migraine has taught me a lot about my personal power. It is a lesson I would have liked to learn another way. Nonetheless, it is mine and it is a painful truth.

I have had migraines since I was in my early 20s, a couple of times a year. When I turned 35, something changed. I had a migraine that lasted four days and I had to go to the hospital before it would stop. I began having episodes four and five days a week and went to a neurologist. He prescribed several medications to bring these headaches under control.

Needless to say, I was pretty much in constant pain, either recovering from a migraine or about to develop one, and my neurologist hadn't really warned me about rebound headache. I was using the medication as prescribed, and I had migraines every week that I could not treat. I was still working full time, in a high-stress job as the executive director of a nonprofit organization, helping people with chronic medical conditions advocate for their needs within the medical system.

The medication was not working well for me. I was still having many migraines, sometimes four to six a week, and sometimes ones that lasted a week, or longer. My physician would adjust the dose, and I would try it again. It still would not work. The pain overwhelmed me, but I accepted it.

As a health educator and patient advocate, I had spent more than 15 years helping people with chronic and life-threatening conditions understand how to get their needs met when dealing with physicians and hospitals. And there I was, in the same position.

I called my doctor during an eight-day migraine and asked for his help. I told him I couldn't live like this anymore. It had been a year and a half, and according to my calculations, I'd had almost 150 migraines. I told him this one was eight days long and I couldn't get rid of it.

You know what he said? "They stop eventually, don't they?"

In a flash, amidst the blinding pain, I figured it out.

I told him, "I can think of a lot of things that eventually go away, but it doesn't mean I should put up with them. You wouldn't tolerate this kind of pain for eight days.

And with that, I fired my doctor.

I found another neurologist with a specialty clinic focused on migraine. She changed my medication, found several triggers in my diet that contributed to my migraines, and in a matter of weeks, cut my headaches in half.

I felt like a new person. It is one thing to be strong for another person when they are ill; it is quite another to find that strength in yourself. I did not realize how much pain I had until it was lifted from me, and in the end, I did not know my own strength until I reflected on my experience and realized what I had endured. ☙

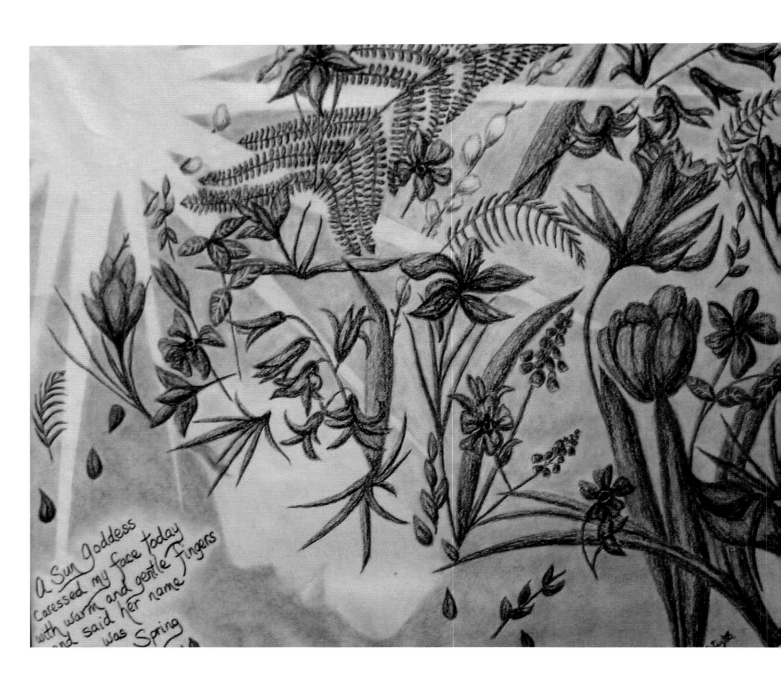

A Sun Goddess
Caressed my face today
with warm and gentle Fingers
and said her name
was Spring

The Other Side of the Tunnel
a victorious journey through migraine pain ©2007

Faith K. Rawley, Age 50, Warrenville, Illinois

when i close my eyes I can still see it all, as if I am watching a replay of a home movie from the 60s, ticking through the life of someone else. But it was my life. It was the life of my family.

I skipped carefully over the cracks in the sidewalk as I clung to my dad's calloused hand. My shiny black patent leather shoes clicked in a hurried rhythm, trying to compete with his long strides. The pleats of my overly starched cotton dress rustled behind us in protest. There would be many of these Sunday marathons throughout my childhood. Our unspoken goal was that together, as a team, we needed to arrive at the arched doorway of our church before the carillon bells reached to the clouds with their final note. It seemed that I was always humming the last stanza of "Amazing Grace" as we reached the threshold of the sanctuary. The majestic oak doors clicked behind us, shutting out the world we left at home. We were now surrounded with stacks of freshly printed bulletins and the expectant smile of a dedicated usher.

The weekly journey to church was a refuge for both of us. Although my dad never verbalized his inner thoughts, (in those days it was not a "manly thing" to do), I could sense his relief. He would let out a deep breathy sigh as we sat in our self-designated balcony pew. Here in our own realm of worship, I knew my dad felt peace. It was a time for him to reflect as he prayerfully requested strength for the days to come. I would lean my tightly curled hair against his arm and notice his freshly dry cleaned suit and the sweet richness of too much Old Spice. On days like these, we depended on each other.

The walk home was always longer. Once we had discussed what I learned in Children's Church and joked about Mrs. Reber's outlandish Sunday hat, we walked in halting silence. My now-dulled shoes dragged in heavy dread. The once-crisp skirt drooped with despair. Our reprieve was over. We both knew our world was about to change back into the inevitable.

My dad leaned into the heavy Victorian door as it begrudgingly welcomed us home. His comment was always the same. "Now remember not to slam it shut. Mom is still sleeping," he tenderly reminded me. "Why don't you go check on her and I will start some lunch." I tiptoed up the weary maple stairway, trying to avoid the creak spots. As I opened my parents' bedroom door, the sun from the hallway window shot through the darkness like a rude intruder. Although she had covered her face with a pillow, I could hear my mother's light breathing. The effects from the Darvon would last for a few hours. For now she was numbed to the constant stabbing pains in her head. The nausea had passed. The serenity of her deep slumber caused me to be happy for her. Earlier that morning, I had lain in the bright pink cocoon of my own bed and cringed at the sounds of her moaning. I squeezed my eyes shut, trying to block out the familiar image of her elegant face creased with agony. At the age of five, I was already accustomed to the tunnel of torment my mother endured with migraine headaches.

Our family braved each storm with her. The routine was the same. Her cheerful deep chestnut brown eyes would become pinched with pain. As the day progressed, her world began to spin. And so did ours. My mother would retreat to the sanctity of a darkened bedroom where grey wool blankets guarded the windows, forbidding any sunlight. Debilitating nausea forced frequent trips down the hall to the bathroom until she could no longer make that trip. A towel or bedside bucket took its place. My dad's boundless patience was only one of the many ways he showed his deep love for my mom. He would automatically administer the waiting prescription of Darvon until I was old enough to read the dosage and watch the clock. Sometimes the migraine pain was so severe that my mother would lie in bed with a brick placed on her forehead. She said the concrete pressure relieved some of the pain. Soon she would alternate with a cool cloth and heating pad. After a day or so, she was ready to eat. Her first craving was always for a baked potato and lemon lime soda. When she was able to communicate once again, she always apologized for what she "put us through." Yet, it was not what "I went through" that stabbed at my soul. My open wound was the helplessness of watching her journey through agony over and over again, not being able to break the cycle. Migraine pain shatters the psyche of its victims and crushes the hearts of loved ones as they watch the struggle for survival in this vortex of agony.

Years passed and our family chartered through the voyage of living with mother's migraines. Carefully made family plans were frequently changed. Sometimes we marched forward as scheduled with one parent at the helm. But most often, we stayed home just to be together. After the storm had passed, we would put another episode of darkness behind us and move forward, until the next time.

Before long I became my mother's caregiver during her painful pilgrimages, occasionally staying home from school to watch over her. When I packed my sack lunch in the morning, I would study her face. Through the billows of steam from her coffee mug, I could determine if it was going to be a good day or not. On the "not" days I would run home from the bus stop to be sure she was in bed and had not taken too many painkillers. Eventually, my mother's level of pain exceeded the strength of a typical dosage. She began to "double up." I became very adept at counting how many red and gray capsules were in the amber bottle before I left for school and recounted to compare in the afternoon. Her life was a constant race, pounding on to keep ahead of piercing migraines. I was a spectator, attending every event and cheering silently for her to keep running. I did not want my mother to come in last.

Despite the expectancy of frequent pain, my mother's migraines did not define who she was. Rather, this anguish forced her to rise above her illness. My mom was one of the most vibrant, artistic, humorous and loving women I have ever met. Her ingenuity brought our family out of many a financial crisis. In a society where it was unheard of for a mother to work outside the home, my mom stepped out in front way before her time. She brought her career to her family. Attending night school for interior design, she honed her given ability for color, texture and style. She followed her education by starting her own business. My mother, the entrepreneur, opened a floral design and antique shop on the first floor of our home. Her business blossomed and buyers drove from suburbs away just to purchase one of her custom made floral arrangements. My heart swelled with pride. She was MY mother.

Amid becoming a successful business woman, my mom suffered for 30 years before finding a doctor who led her to the end of her oppressive migraines. In addition to discovering that my mom had many food allergies, this miraculous physician also found her thyroid to be underactive. He prescribed thyroxin and a carefully guarded diet. From that point on, my mother was no longer held captive by the chains of migraine headaches. My mom was 45 years old when she began to live life without the foreboding agony of migraines.

It would be expected to conclude this story with a typical happy ending by stating, "I finally saw my mom for the beautiful woman she really was." But that would be false.

I always saw my mother's beauty. I grew up seeing her radiance in some way every day, even during the jaded ones. As parents, we often scrutinize every second of our childrearing skills. Guilt for things done, or not done, become a quagmire which consumes us in negativity. Perhaps many would label the documentary of my childhood with a mixed review of neglect and growing up too quickly. Yet, those feelings are not in my box of memories. Was it a difficult time? I would be remiss to not admit the road was rocky. But what family, or person, does not walk through ominous tunnels in life's journey? It is how those difficult paths are navigated that makes all the difference in the destination. A base of hope and faith charts the course in the right direction.

Despite her illness, my mother taught me and loved me. I felt her respond when I reached into her depths of pain and held out my hand. I learned compassion. I observed her persevere and pray as she faced seemingly insurmountable mountains. I learned about fortitude and faith in God. My mother encouraged me to be confident and become who I was created to be. Watching and loving her helped me to grow into the woman I am today.

My mom has now passed into an eternity void of any kind of suffering. But not before she had an opportunity to live three more decades without a migraine. She will always remain in my heart and memory, a very integral part of my own journey. Not remembered as someone who spent part of her life in a treacherous tunnel of pain. But as the loving wife, mother, grandmother, friend and creative woman who kept walking steadfastly until she found the end of her dismal tunnel. She made it through. With grace and dignity, my mother found the other side. ❧

The First Time
©2007

Amethyst Hawkins
Age 27
Portland, Oregon

11 years old,
the first time
finding
something
wronging in me

11 years old, and
stricken with unknowness
I can only see half
of the sky
half of a father
half
of me

11 years old,
curious child faces
peering
through this thickness
and
finding me there
all muted, abandoned
and
crashing

11 years old
and discovering
something wronging
in me
for the first
time

years go by,
I find myself surviving
again
and again and
growing the idea that
maybe
this
special burden
has been given me

like a gift that
takes years
to unwrap
some
unfathomed relationship
to death or
simply
silence

because
upon resurfacing,
that first breath
of air
is like sweet afternoon sun
in my veins

it says
you have overcome,
you are alive my dear
and living
for the first time

see your wings?

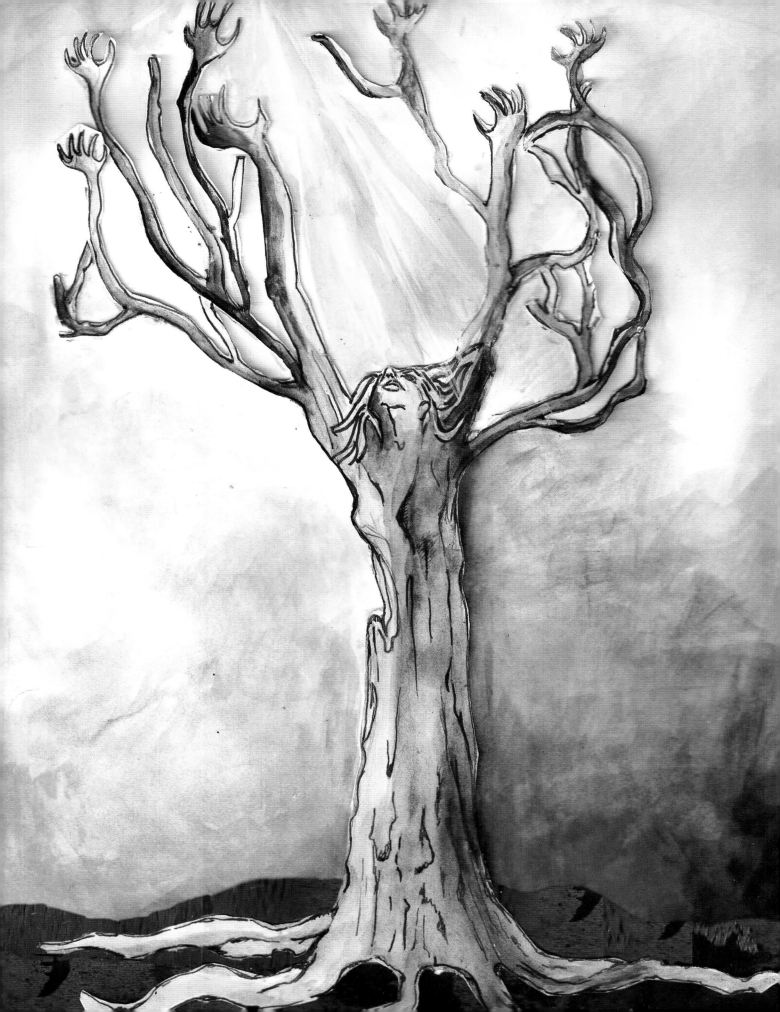

Storm ©2007

beneath the storm
into the void
i
fall
dreaming of peace

Rebekah Jorgensen
Age 25, St. Paul, Minnesota

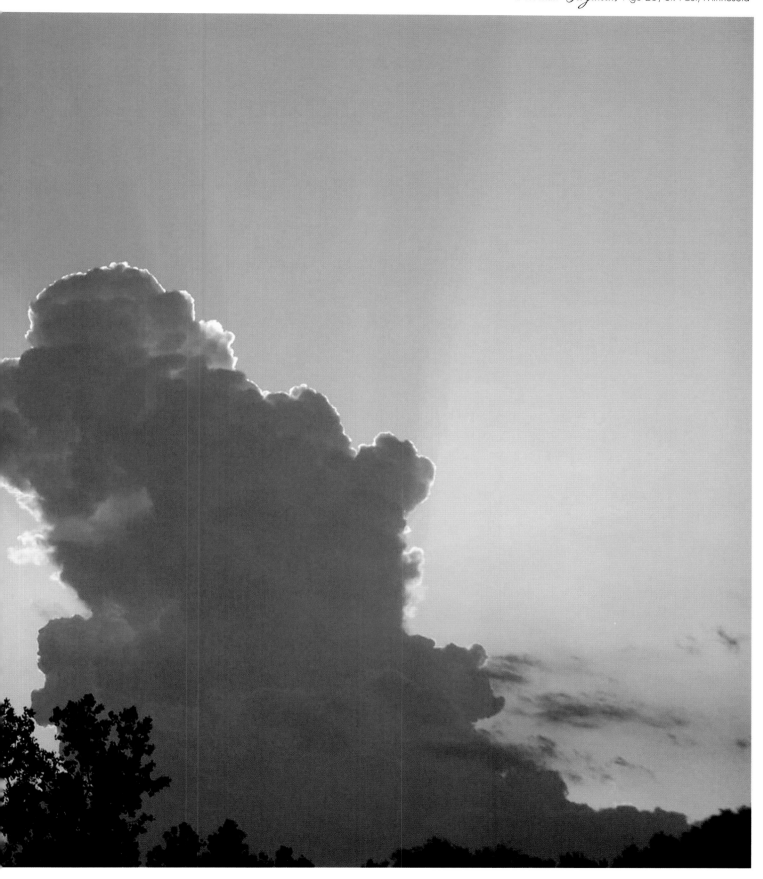

The Gift
of Migraine
©2007

Lauren Koblara
Age 26
West Brookfield, Massachusetts

There are days when I wake up without pain. No lingering sensitivity to light, no twitching muscles at my temples, no pressure behind my eyes. When a day like this comes along, I am sure to take notice. I wake up determined to make this "good day" an event.

Most chronic migraine sufferers know what I am talking about. When the majority of your days are spent noticing auras, fighting off pain, and finally feeling the aftermath of migraine, you tend to hold pain-free days on a pedestal. My pain-free days bring out a manic side of myself. I am thrilled with the concept of a full day. I make lists and accomplish as much as possible, enjoying every trivial aspect of everyday life. Pain-free days are something to be cherished.

I was about three years old when my mother noticed there was something wrong. She'd come home from work and find me with my face wedged between the couch cushions, blanket over my head. When she brought me to the doctor's office, they told her it was allergies, gave me a prescription and sent us on our merry way. One day I was having one of these "allergy headaches" while at preschool and had a seizure-like episode. It was after this episode that I was diagnosed with cluster headaches. I was never offered any kind of treatment that I can recall. Maybe there was no magic pill back then, but I remember having to take children's Tylenol and Benadryl and just sleeping it off.

As I grew older, the cluster headaches evolved into migraines and I still wasn't offered any real treatment. When I was about 16, I had a migraine so bad that my poor Grandmother was sure that I was having an aneurism. She called a neighbor, who thankfully was a doctor, and I got an emergency prescription for migraine meds. The meds certainly knocked me out, but it was much better than trying not to move and praying for death. A few short months later, I read about triptan drugs like Imitrex. The idea of stopping a migraine dead in its tracks made me giddy. I marched into my next doctor's appointment and demanded a prescription. She determined that I was a good fit for the drug and wrote a script for me. I have since gone through a few different kinds of migraine meds trying to find what works best, but I am so thankful that these treatments are out there and that they work for me. They are one of the miracles in my life.

Still, there is something to be said for a day that can simply be lived. The rarity of days like that makes them precious. They are the back-handed gift of Migraine. My journey through migraines has led me to appreciate a good day. Even if it is something as small as household chores, I know I can accomplish them better on a day without a migraine. Days like those come and I don't know what to do first. I scramble to get together with friends and family, to go outside and work in the garden, to read the book that has sat on my nightstand under heating pads and cold eye packs. Simple things that most people take for granted as part of their daily grind become a celebration of what I can achieve when I feel well.

I admit it is a challenge to keep a positive attitude when I am blinded by pain and can barely stand, and I sometimes struggle with keeping things in perspective. My pain may be chronic and at times debilitating, but I have the promise of better days in my future and the support of people around me. I know that sandwiched between some mediocre days I will experience one of those extraordinary gifts... a good day. ❧

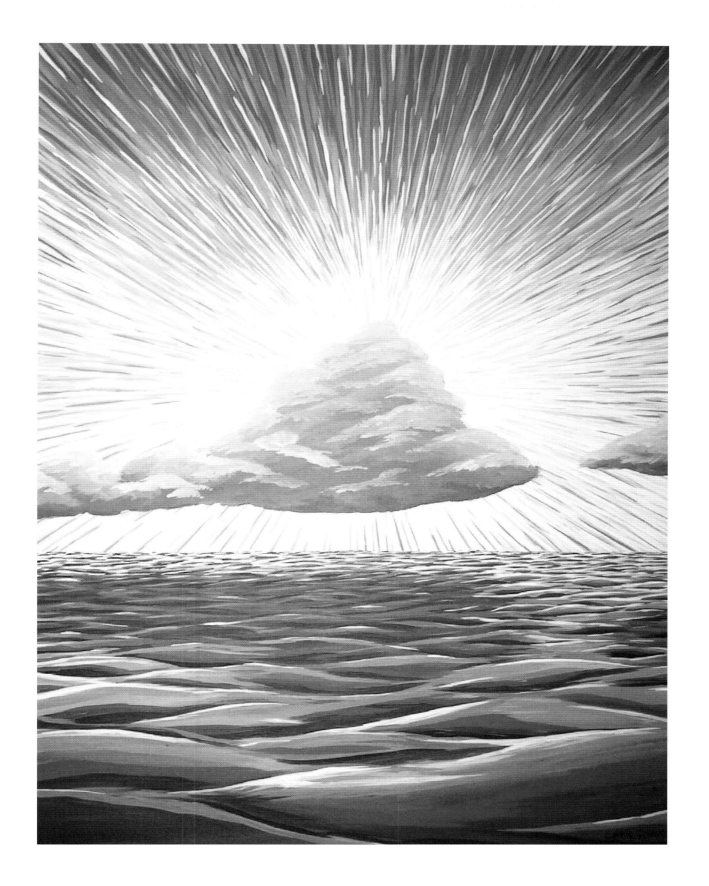

HEAVENLY LIGHT ©2007
Cedric Colond, Ottawa, Ontario, Canada

The pain of migraines resembles an intense storm. Frozen in time, one moment perceived as eternity.
The clouds pass with a gentle breeze and warm light, the integrity of the soul tested and perseveres.

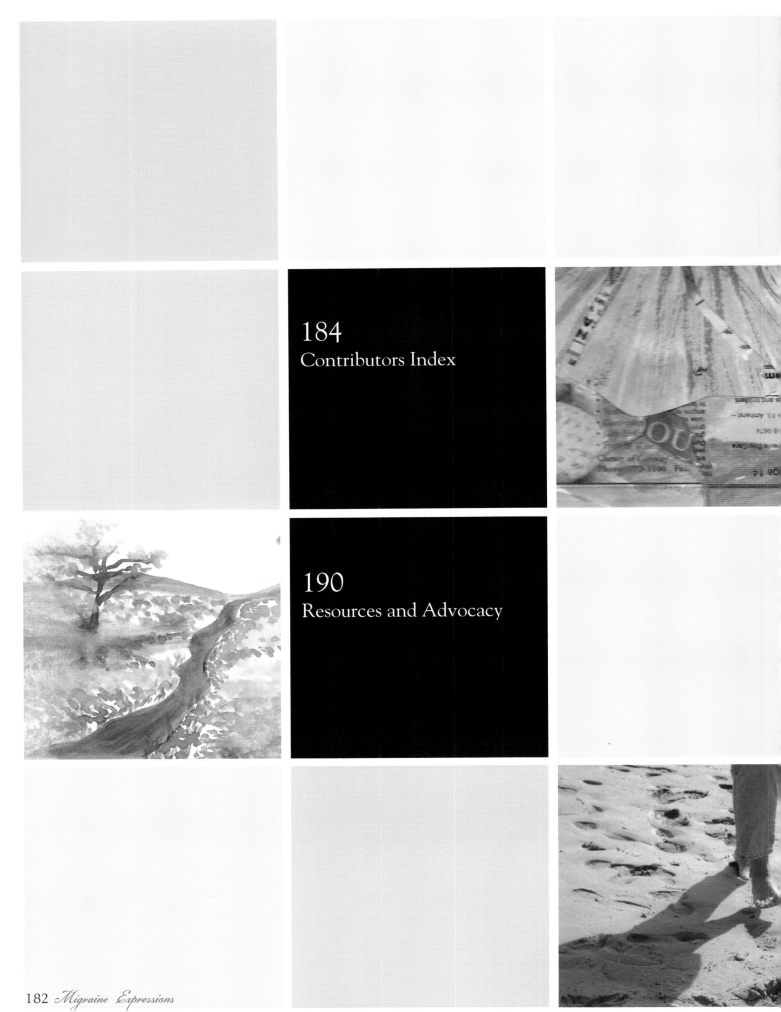

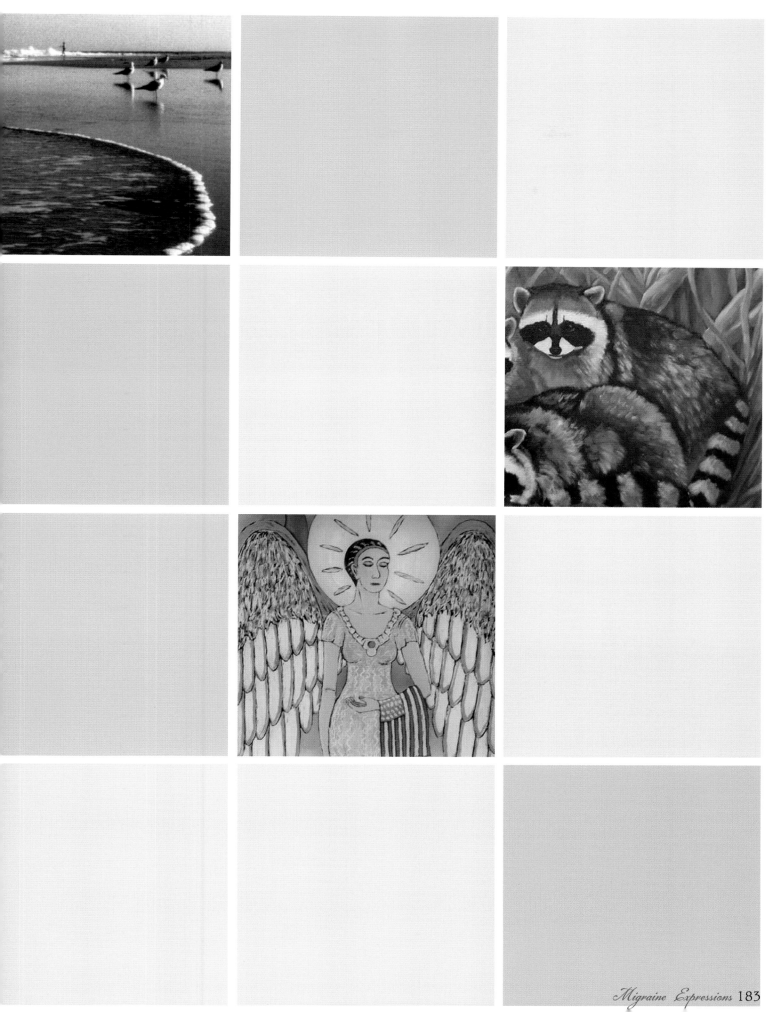

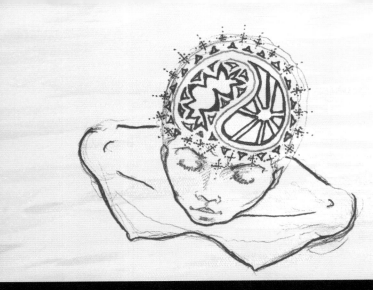

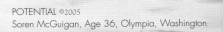

POTENTIAL ©2005
Soren McGuigan, Age 36, Olympia, Washington

CONTRIBUTORS *Index*

continued on page 186

continued on page 188

Eric Ding, of Boston, Massachusetts, and currently a postdoctoral fellow at the Harvard School of Public Health and a med student at the Boston University School of Medicine, contributed several migraine background articles and quotes as well as much appreciated support and enthusiasm for this project.

RESOURCES & *Advocacy*

MIGRAINE/HEADACHE ORGANIZATIONS WORLDWIDE (ALPHABETICAL)

ACHE (American Headache Society Committee for Headache Education), www.achenet.org

American Headache Society, www.americanheadachesociety.org

City of London Migraine Clinic, www.colmc.org.uk

European Headache Federation, www.ehf-org.org

Headache Network Canada, www.headachenetwork.ca

International Headache Society, www.i-h-s.org

M.A.G.N.U.M., National Migraine Association www.migraines.org

Migraine Action Association, www.migraine.org.uk

Migraine Trust, The, www.migrainetrust.org

National Headache Foundation, www.headaches.org

World Headache Alliance, www.w-h-a.org

MIGRAINE AND HEADACHE ADVOCACY AND RESEARCH SITES

Alliance for Headache Disorders Advocacy, www.allianceforheadacheadvocacy.org

Lifting the Burden, www.l-t-b.org

Migraine Research Foundation, www.migraineresearchfoundation.org

We Are Advocates, Teri Robert, www.weareadvocates.com

INFORMATIONAL SITES, BLOGS, AND FORUMS

Abi's Migrainous Wanderings, Abigail Addison, http://abimigraines.blogspot.com

Cleveland Clinic Center for Headache and Pain, http://cms.clevelandclinic.org/neuroscience

Diamond Headache Clinic, www.diamondheadache.com

Down the Rabbit Hole: The journey of a migraineur, http://a-migraineur.blogspot.com

Headache & Migraine News Blog, James Cottrill, http://blog.relieve-migraine-headache.com

Help for Headaches & Migraine, Teri Robert, www.helpforheadaches.com

Help for Headaches, G. Brent Lucas, www.headache-help.org, Canada

Jefferson Headache Center, www.jefferson.edu/headache

Life in the Canadian Desert, Jackie Taylor, www.jackietaylorsblog.blogspot.com

Mayo Clinic, www.mayoclinic.com

Michigan Head-Pain & Neurological Institute, www.mhni.com

Migraine Chick, http://migrainechickie.blogspot.com

My Migraine Connection, The Health Central Network, www.healthcentral.com/migraine

New England Center for Headache, www.headachenech.com

New York Times' Migraine Blog, http://migraine.blogs.nytimes.com

Robbins Headache Clinic, www.headachedrugs.com

Somebody Heal Me, Diana E. Lee, http://somebodyhealme.dianalee.net

The Daily Headache, Kerrie Smyres, www.thedailyheadache.com

The Headache Center of Southern California, www.the-headachecenter.com

The Migraine Girl, Janet Geddis, http://themigrainegirl.blogspot.com

Weathering Migraine Storms, http://deborah-weatheringmigrainestorms.blogspot.com

SITES WITH MIGRAINE ART AND OR POETRY

ACHE (American Headache Society Committee for Headache Education), www.achenet.org

Migraine Action Association, http://www.migraine.org.uk/competition.aspx

Migraine Action Association, Children's Web site, www.migraine4kids.org.uk/creative.htm

Migraine Aura Foundation, www.migraine-aura.org

National Headache Foundation, www.headaches.org

Ronda's Migraine Page, http://www.migrainepage.com/images.html

Editor's Note: This list is by no means all-inclusive, and once you begin searching you will readily find many additional helpful Web sites and blogs. Please remember to confirm information found on the Internet by consulting several sources.

continued on page 192

Tribute

No recognition
No honor
No glory
No gain
For your pain
Your suffering
Your sacrifice

No envy
No admiration
No desire
No awe
For your skill
Your wisdom
Your expertise

No army
No troops
No teammates
No allied brigades
For your struggle
Your fight
Your war

No laurels
No badges
No accolades
No standing ovations
For your courage
Your resolve
Your feats

You always win. Every time, you beat.
You are a warrior, a champion.
I am your fan.
Today,
Every day,
I am proud of you.

Kelly Jo Blondin ©2008
Age 23, Montara, California